Medi-Cross III

50 Advanced Medical Terminology Crossword Puzzles

for Medical, Pre-Med, Nursing, Chiropractic, EMTs, PTs and Other Health Care Professionals and Crossword Lovers

John McLeod

Introduction

Medi-Cross III is another collection with new puzzles and more medical terms. It is intended for those looking to increase their vocabulary in the fields of science relating to the human body and for those interested in etymology and linguistics.

The Medi-Cross series remain the only American-style crossword books containing over 70 medical terms in each puzzle, making them ideal for those focused on this area of knowledge and expertise.

1

Across

1. ____sthesia; pain sense
5. Medicinal agent vehicle
11. ___umen; earwax
14. Inferences from the truth
15. Relating to the tongue undersurface
16. ____tic; relating to syphilis
17. Condition of being blocked
19. Insulin-like growth factor (abbrev)
20. To pull something back
21. A line of equal retinal sensitivity in the visual field
23. ____flexia; lack of reflexes
24. Dacarbazine (abbrev)
26. Unit of perceived loudness
27. ____flexion; upward foot movement
29. Rib ____; skeletal thorax
32. Rainbow-like eye part
33. Intermittent acute porphyria (abbrev)
35. ____phobia; fear of light flashes
37. A disease of tropical fishes
38. The total of the stages of an organisms life
41. Familial adenomatous polyposis (abbrev)
43. Prefix meaning 'within'
44. Cumulative trauma disorders (abbrev)
45. ____roid; resembling a dream
47. Reproductive cell of females
49. ____osis; programmed cell death
53. ____osis; exaggerated lumbar curve
54. ____icemia; blood poisoning
56. Counterimmunoelectrophoresis (abbrev)
57. Cavity filling substance
61. Tooth with three cusps
63. ____gut; suture material
64. Medial epicondyle of humerus
66. ____ectomy; removal of the ileum
67. The vertebral column
68. ____ine; an amino acid
69. ____ophobia; fear of disease
70. Prefix referring to vision
71. Hairs

Down

1. Directed away from the mouth
2. ____motor; relating to voluntary movements
3. Stomach (Greek)
4. ____ogen; female sex hormone
5. ____ation; belching
6. Referring to milk
7. ___egumentary; relating to the skin
8. Roman 13
9. ____emia; inositol in the blood
10. ____genic; originating in the kidney
11. Erectile female sex organ
12. Referring to controlled procreation
13. To renew
18. To send out
22. 23rd letter of the Greek alphabet
25. Cheeselike
28. The breaking of a moral law
30. ___eric; nonspecific, common
31. ____tive; not essential
34. ____phobia; fear of overworking
36. Unsteady; unstable
38. Performs a surgical procedure
39. Gastric dilatation and volvulus (abbrev)
40. Inosine 5-diphosphate (abbrev)
41. Folic acid
42. Prefix meaning 'irregular'
46. Intermediate density lipoprotein (abbrev)
48. Relating to a measuring system
50. Simple eyes of insects
51. _____ gland; epiphysis celebri
52. _____genous; causing lockjaw
55. ____plasia; abnormal differentiation of tissue
58. Prefix meaning 'old age'
59. Acetaminophen (abbrev)
60. ____urate; to urinate
62. Dihydroxyacetone phosphate (abbrev)
65. ___emia; sulfur in blood

2

Across

1. _____ism; lack of pigment
6. 5-lipooxygenase activating protein (acronym)
10. Excitatory postsynaptic potential (abbrev)
14. _____lagnia; sexual attraction toward prostitutes
15. _____sis; abnormal hunger
16. Frequency that an event occurs per unit of time
17. Physical maltreatment
18. Acute sensory axonal motor neuropathy (abbrev)
19. _____nal; everlasting
20. Surgical fixation
21. _____pathy; disease of the viscera
23. Blood-sucking arachnid parasites
25. Directly observed therapy (abbrev)
26. Prefix meaning 'hearing'
29. Prefix referring to the brain enveloping membrane
33. ___tropics; brain enhancers
34. _____tid; neck artery
37. Acronym for as low as reasonably achievable
38. Regeneration of bone
42. Sharp momentary pain
43. Dacarbazine (abbrev)
44. ___lingus; sexual stimulation of the anus
45. Young child learning to walk
47. Burns with hot liquid
50. ___ectomy; surgical removal of the penis
51. Acute zonal occult outer retinopathy (abbrev)
53. Concretion in the gallbladder
57. Pertaining to the first portion of the large bowel
61. Nitrogenous endproduct of protein metabolism
62. Expiratory positive airway pressure (abbrev)
63. Hornlike projection
64. _____itis; inflammation of an opening
65. Repose after exertion
66. _____ment; the longitudinal position of a limb
67. Free from harm
68. _____geny; development of an organism
69. Vulvar folds

Down

1. Acetaminophen (abbrev)
2. A curved or rounded projection
3. _____ism; spasmodic grinding of the teeth
4. Confined to the site of origin (2 words)
5. Cognition
6. A small, glass receptacle
7. Mispronounces the sibilants S and Z
8. _____gam; cavity filler
9. Waxy substance used to style hair
10. Capable of becoming rigid
11. _____ology; study of disease
12. _____osis; a bodily passage narrowing
13. _____melia; congenital deformity of the limbs
22. Occurring on the 9th day
24. The source of cocaine
26. _____osis; failure of ossification
27. ___genic; arising from a rib
28. A ripe ovum
29. _____lalia; pathological speech problem
30. Pertaining to the nose
31. To reduce to powder
32. Suffix meaning 'a disease process resulting therefrom'
35. _____ology; study of men's health
36. Disease-spreading rodent
39. The flattened end of a motor neuron
40. Eyes provocatively
41. Enteric cytopathogenic swine orphan (abbrev)
46. _____lith; intestinal calculus
48. Relating to spheroid bacteria
49. Small cavity within a tissue
51. _____omosis; blood vessel coalescence
52. Prefix signifying one sextillionth
53. Gingivae
54. Part of a surface
55. _____let; a layer of phospholipid
56. Not obstructed
58. A baby's bed
59. _____itis; blood vessel inflammation
60. ___tic; mentally ill person

3

Across

1. Warms
6. ____algia; leg pain
10. Illuminating device
14. Group of eight
15. ____phobia; fear of being poisoned
16. Rainbow-like eye part
17. Removal of the gallbladder
20. A specific point in time
21. Enzootic
22. Referring to the ankle
25. ____noid; weblike
26. ____pedic; clubfooted
30. ____otic; fetus-surrounding fluid
32. 3rd stage of nucleus division in mitosis
35. Roman 890
41. Congenital absence of the brain
43. Visible evidence of a disease
44. Muscle protein which influences tropomyosin to initiate contraction
45. ____myosarcoma; malignant tumor of the uterus muscle
47. Prefix meaning toward or on the left side
48. Pertaining to birds
53. Pertaining to the nose
56. To undergo tissue death
58. Resembling a mole or birthmark
63. Between the transverse processes of the vertebrae
66. Render unconscious by cerebral trauma
67. A chill or fit of shivering
68. The most prominent craniometric point at the occipital protuberance
69. Bones
70. ____genous; originating in cheese
71. Examinations

Down

1. High osmolar contrast medium (abbrev)
2. Sound repetition
3. Smallest unit of an element
4. Prefix meaning 'over a distance'
5. A mold for keeping a skin graft in place
6. External hordeolum
7. Chief of Staff (abbrev)
8. Nonresident graduate who assists in medical care
9. Spleen
10. Metric unit of capacity
11. An agreeable odor
12. To imitate or simulate
13. ____ology; science of mind and behavior
18. Computed tomography angiography (abbrev)
19. Canadian dental grp.
23. To treat with a light beam device
24. Severe intellectual disability
26. Elicits a tendon reflex
27. ____omy; body structure study
28. ____ary; adapted for tearing
29. Isopropylthiogalactoside (abbrev)
31. ____phobia; fear of different mental conceptions
33. ____string; posterior knee tendon
34. ____eptic; nervous system stimulant
36. Community psychiatry program (abbrev)
37. ____uria; presence of bile in the blood
38. Walking stick
39. Roman forty-four
40. ____phobia; fear of dogs
42. Contralateral routing of signal (abbrev)
46. The capacity to do work
48. ____coria; asymmetric pupils
49. Outlets that discharges pus
50. A sudden attack
51. ____virus; disease transmitted by rodents
52. ____epinephrine; a vasoconstrictor
54. Autonomic nervous system (abbrev)
55. ____ation; support on a cushion of air
57. With no delay
59. ____section; phlebotomy
60. Fetor ____; halitosis
61. ____onic; having equal tension
62. A toothlike structure
64. ____iform; ear-shaped
65. ____natal; newborn

Across

1. ____uria; rapid urine excretion during fasting
5. Unable to hear
9. Lip-shaped structures
14. Principles or rules
15. Roman 1041
16. Relating to the inion
17. Pertaining to ileum and cecum
19. A growth protruding from a mucous membrane
20. Small vascular processes
21. ____form; resembling a network
23. A quantity of matter
24. Increase in size
26. ____uria; blood in the urine
28. ____phobia; fear of involuntarily shaking
30. Greater omentum
33. Treat with a light beam device
36. Small mass of foreign cells
38. ____pelvis; twisted pelvis
39. Emergency Medical Technician (abbrev)
40. A monosaccharide containing five carbon atoms
42. ____iculation; joint
43. A delimited area
45. Any weblike tissue
46. ____psoas; hip flexor
47. Enlarged and inflamed lymph nodes
49. Tunica ____; middle artery wall layer
51. Passage leading into a cavity
53. Implying nearness to the corpus callosum
57. ____atry; study and treatment of speech disorders
59. Acronym for p-aminobenzoic acid
61. ____genic; appetite stimulating
62. ____lysis; decomposition of uric acid
64. Inflammation of entire ear
66. ____encephalia; absence of the cerebellum
67. Human diploid cell vaccine (abbrev)
68. Acronym for contralateral routing of signal
69. ____genic; starch-forming
70. Prefix meaning oil
71. ____motor; related to movements caused by sound

Down

1. Oval eminence on medulla oblongata
2. ____opsia; visual perseveration
3. To increase in size
4. To separate
5. Director of Medical Education (abbrev)
6. Feces
7. Winglike structures
8. Dirtiness
9. Labium
10. Prefix meaning 'irregular'
11. Pertaining to both sides
12. Light beams
13. Acrocephalosyndactyly (abbrev)
18. ____hosis; liver disorder
22. Isoelectric point (abbrev)
25. Biological unit of heredity
27. Insect parasite that causes scabies
29. ____pyesis; suppuration in bone
31. ____form; shaped like a leather bottle
32. ____toxin; a food poison
33. ____ianism; sapphism
34. ____tate; cut off
35. Condition of being resistant to change
37. The ability to endure a stimulus
40. To remove the outer layer by stripping
41. Prefix meaning 'delight in cruelty'
44. Resembling a cone in shape
46. Medical practice specialties (suffix)
48. ____sis; toxic condition
50. ____onic; having equal tension
52. ____phobia; fear of being buried alive
54. ____grade; moving backward
55. The brain and spinal cord
56. ____trichic; having straight hair
57. ____tic; mentally ill person
58. Active range of motion (abbrev)
60. Basic activities of daily living (abbrev)
63. ____matomania; abnormal impulse to dwell on certain words
65. ____cyte; egg cell

5

Across
1. _____omosis; blood vessel coalescence
6. Short sleeps
10. _____otomy; incision into an apical structure
14. _____geal; of the tailbone
15. _____omy; body structure study
16. _____toxin; a food poison
17. Paralysis of the isthmus faucium
20. A measured quantity of a drug
21. _____algia; referred pain
22. Stand firm against
23. Roman 1059
25. Bed covering for administering oxygen
26. _____osis; arrested action of the sebaceous glands
29. Any disorder of pregnancy
33. Chimpanzee coryza agent (abbrev)
34. Internal layer of protective material
36. _____ crest; pelvic ridge
37. A specified period of time
39. Walking sticks
41. Ethylenediaminetetraacetic acid (abbrev)
42. _____nia; sleep difficulty
44. To perceive flavour in the mouth
46. Estrogen replacement therapy (abbrev)
47. Newborn
49. _____genes; related to the eyebrows
51. _____oid; pencil-like
52. Dimethyl sulfoxide (abbrev.)
53. Stomach
56. _____tus; an opening
57. Antibody-dependent cell-mediated cytotoxicity (abbrev.)
61. Directed from front to back
64. A tubular passage
65. Residue remaining after percolation of a drug
66. Qualitative or quantitative analysis of a substance
67. Method of reducing pain by electric current (abbrev)
68. _____genic; idiopathic
69. _____phobia; proctophobia

Down
1. A proton donor
2. _____mania; hypochondriacism
3. Performs
4. A systematic plan of action
5. _____panic; resonant
6. Scalp area just below the occipital protuberance
7. _____eptic; nervous system stimulant
8. _____amnesia; false recollection
9. Looks intently
10. Absence of a heart beat
11. _____form; pea-shaped wrist bone
12. Inflammation of (suffix)
13. _____algia; rib pain
18. Pertaining to ear inflammation
19. _____form; lens-shaped
24. _____iatry; study and treatment of speech disorders
25. _____ major; arm adductor
26. Muscle protein localized in the I band of myofibrils
27. Exhibition of questionable behavior
28. Prefix referring to the ankle
29. Relating to the cheek
30. _____osis; hyperferremia
31. Medical practice specialty (suffix)
32. _____phagy; the eating of excrement
35. Pertaining to birth
38. Grotesquely abnormal beings
40. _____algia; mouth pain
43. Dura _____; outer brain and spinal cord membrane
45. Exophthalmos-producing substance (abbrev)
48. A caseous tumor
50. Having a noisy voice
52. _____pathy; intervertebral cartilage disease
53. A manner of walking
54. _____brachium; forearm
55. _____osis; a bodily passage narrowing
56. A head projection on various animals
58. A round flat plate
59. The outer covering of an organ
60. _____lysis; destruction by cold
62. Periaqueductal gray (abbrev)
63. Hearing organ

6

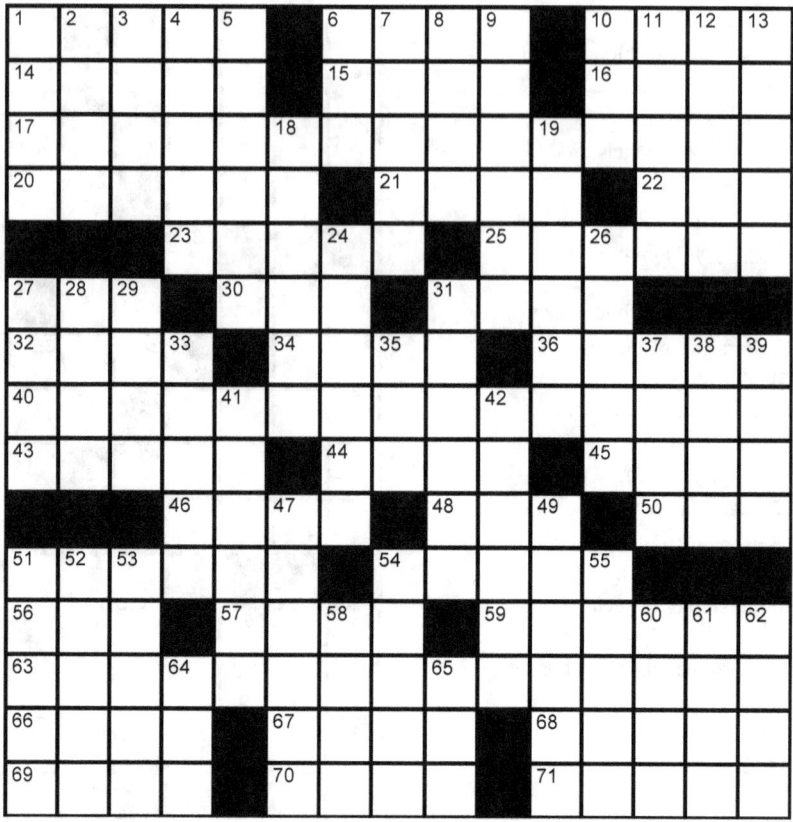

Across
1. Upper heart chambers
6. Cricohyoidoepiglottopexy (abbrev)
10. Excitatory postsynaptic potential (abbrev)
14. _____rrhea; drooling
15. _____dynia; sinew pain
16. _____xeny; change of host by a parasite
17. Between the collarbones
20. _____lysis; fat emulsion in the digestive process
21. Dissolution (prefix)
22. Roman 1002
23. Mispronounces the sibilants S and Z
25. _____genesis; the origin and development of organs
27. ___ate; moonlike wrist bone
30. Computed tomography angiography (abbrev)
31. _____genesis; origin and growth of a neoplasm
32. Other licensed antifungal therapies (abbrev)
34. Acetaminophen (abbrev)
36. Lip-shaped structures
40. Within the epithelial cells
43. Nostril
44. Presence in urine (suffix)
45. _____oid; pencil-like
46. Performs
48. Community psychiatry program (abbrev)
50. ___tropia; cross-eye
51. Condition of listlessness and a form of melancholia
54. Muscle contraction neuron
56. Chronic respiratory disease (abbrev)
57. Prefix signifying one trillion
59. Agent that induces vomitting
63. Study of body divisions (2 wds)
66. _____dotal; based on case histories

67. Inspiratory positive airway pressure (abbrev)
68. A two-footed conjoined twin
69. Treat with a light beam
70. _____genesis; the formation of gas
71. _____osis; bone mass within a bone

Down
1. Lateral attachment of inguinal ligament (abbrev)
2. A shade of a color
3. Frequency that an event occurs per unit of time
4. Pertaining to the distal small intestine
5. Referring to the main heart artery
6. Cytotoxic T lymphocytes (abbrev)
7. Restores to health
8. Desire to have another's qualities for oneself

9. Substance that is injurious to health
10. Medicinal Australian bird oil
11. Under surface of the foot
12. To dye
13. _____mania; impulse to wander away from home
18. Ribs
19. _____ of Willis; anastomosis of the brain
24. The first downy growth of beard
26. Objectives an organism seeks to attain
27. Lumbus
28. Medial forearm bone
29. _____emia; presence of sodium in blood
31. Prefix referring to vision
33. A group of three associated entities
35. Gaseous mixture in the atmosphere
37. Sieze with the teeth

38. Light beams
39. _____path; traditional doctor
41. _____genous; producing hydroperitoneum
42. Incomplete antigen
47. Ribbonlike band of tissue
49. A waxy substance used to style hair
51. Affecting the extremities
52. A V-shaped cut
53. Surface borders
54. _____ bone; zygoma
55. _____itis; inflammation of the optomeninx
58. A sexual assault
60. _____phobia; fear of certain places
61. Most inferior of several similar structures
62. Enclosed, fluid-filled sac
64. ___ pack; cold local application
65. ___neurosis; sheet-like tendinous expansion

Across

1. A solemn declaration
5. Incapable of normal locomotion
9. Small openings into hollow organs
14. ____form; ear-shaped
15. A mental conception
16. ____born; born dead
17. Freezing of a body part
19. Any anatomic bandlike structure
20. A pouch
21. ____tectomy; removal of the liver
22. Vessel in which substances are ground with a pestle
23. ____phobia; fear of religious or sacred objects
25. Quantity of drug to be taken
26. ____dynia; pain in the penis
28. Recurring regularly
32. ____purulent; characterized by bloody pus
33. Bubbling sounds in the lungs
34. Isonicotinic acid hydrazide (abbrev)
35. ____geny; development of an organism
36. Denatures
37. ____form; resembling bone
38. ___noid; gland-like
39. A taste bud
40. Outer; external
41. Sunstroke
43. Stretch out
44. Other licensed antifungal therapies (abbrev)
45. Pertaining to birds
46. Toward the tail
49. ____thesia; lack of sensation
50. ___emia; sulfur in the blood
53. Epitympanic recess
54. The tip of the anterior nasal spine
56. Anterior part of the thorax
57. A small mass of foreign cells
58. Clavus
59. ____phrodite; person with intersexuality
60. Female breasts (slang)
61. ____pagus; twins joined at the occiput

Down

1. Big, clumsy people
2. Pre-migraine sensation
3. Bone elevation of proximal femur
4. Belonging to a male
5. ____motor; relating to voluntary movements
6. ____cyte; fat cell
7. Prefix meaning 'beyond' or 'after'
8. Experimental allergic encephalitis (abbrev)
9. Bone formation; ossification
10. ____cilia; non-motile microvilli
11. A shade of a color
12. ____cus; hip flexor
13. Like a wing
18. ____rrhagia; hemorrhage from the nipple
22. The accepted traditional customs of society
24. ____psoas; hip flexor
25. A triangular shape
26. Ilio____; thigh flexor
27. ____capped; disabled
28. Concave parts of the hands
29. The act of expanding
30. ____itary; injurious to health
31. A youth
33. To become less severe for a time
36. Toward the median plane of the body
37. Prefix meaning 'eight'
39. _____crasia; abnormal composition of mother's milk
40. To have life
42. Poisoning by iodine
43. Specific occurrences
45. ____omosis; blood vessel coalescence
46. ____exia; severe state of ill health
47. ____roma; artery wall mass
48. ____itis; inflammation in the womb
49. Angiotensin-converting enzyme inhibitors (abbrev)
51. ____zontal; perpendicular to the vertical
52. ____cent; benign
54. ___acid; acid buffering substance
55. Hydrochloric acid (abbrev)

Across

1. A baby's bed
5. Source of cocaine
9. A holding device
14. ____rrhagia; excessive uterine bleeding
15. Anionic neutrophil-activating peptide (abbrev)
16. Axillary hairs
17. Within the peritoneal cavity
20. Pertaining to a minute infectious agent
21. ____ordination; ataxia
22. ____tid; neck artery
23. Graft versus host reaction (abbrev)
25. ____omy; body structure study
27. Anterior aspect of the head
30. Relating to a small secretory sac
35. Bad cholesterol (abbrev.)
36. Roman 59
37. A ridgelike structure
38. ____virus; disease transmitted by rodents
40. Roman 540
42. Enzyme released by the kidney
43. Restore to the normal state
45. In ____; within the body
47. Electrooculography (abbrev)
48. Inner layer of the retina
50. Walking stick
51. A hemorrhoidal tumor
52. ____pexy; surgical fixation of ileum
54. ____algia; leg pain
57. ____nestic; assisting the memory
59. Ensnares
63. Absence of the cerebellum
66. ____coria; asymmetric pupils
67. ____cent; not harmful
68. ____itis; inflammation of the heart
69. ____phagia; swallowing food without mastication
70. Reduces a fracture
71. ____mania; compulsive shopping

Down

1. Roman 904
2. ____capsule; capsule of the kidney
3. ____insic; of internal origin
4. GLA-rich medicinal herb
5. Cradle ____; infant scalp disease
6. Resembling a dream
7. ____ivore; flesh eating mammal
8. Referring to the tip
9. Carbohydrates (abbrev)
10. A confection
11. Part of a surface
12. Mark left after healing
13. ____motor; moving the hair
18. ____eoli; oxygen exchange pockets
19. Characterized by continuous tension
24. High-frequency ventilation (abbrev.)
26. ____phobia; fear of small skin parasites
27. A gradual tapering or spreading outward
28. ____al; situated near the kidney
29. A fissure or groove
31. Roman 76
32. A narrow ridge or streak on a surface
33. Negatively charged ion
34. The difference between the limits of a variable
36. Prefix referring to tears
39. Tumor
41. Liquid preparation rubbed into the skin
44. Weblike tissues
46. ____late; cup-shaped
49. ____elbow; lateral epicondylitis
50. ____brachialis; arm flexor
53. ____ology; study of animal behavior
54. A short sharp sound
55. ____umption; body wasting
56. ____tropic; directed against the cause
58. Breakout of pimples
60. ____ine; an amino acid
61. ____formis; external hip rotator
62. Delight in cruelty (prefix)
64. ____tropics; brain enhancers
65. ____ology; the science of dosage

Across

1. ____oid; S-shaped
5. Anionic neutrophil-activating peptide (abbrev)
9. _____gram; breast screening procedure
14. Large intestine (prefix)
15. ____topic; occurring at the usual place
16. ____ology; study of dreams
17. Abnormality called "Ghost teeth"
20. ___mus; acidity or alkalinity indicator
21. ___ectasis; collapsed lung
22. Saltlike
23. Outer layer of the iris
25. ____phonia; thick
26. Computed tomography angiography (abbrev)
27. Belonging to a female
28. Canine adenovirus (abbrev)
31. A rib
34. Concave part of the hand
35. ____mania; a longing for a particular food
36. Between two digit bones
39. A tubular passage
40. ____utism; excessive bodily hair
41. An agreeable odor
42. A charged particle
43. The germinated and dried seed of barley
44. ___tic; syphilitic
45. ____pharynx; superior portion of the pharynx
46. Channel
50. Dwarfishness
53. A people
54. ___ognosis; the understanding of speech
55. Facial neuralgia caused by a decayed tooth
58. _____dynia; breast pain
59. ____form; resembling bone
60. Consumes
61. _____algia; joint pain
62. _____ cell; any precursor cell
63. A nuisance

Down

1. _____coid; wormlike
2. Relating to iodine
3. _____is; vocal apparatus of the larynx
4. ___aural; relating to one ear
5. Congenital absence of the external ears
6. Small round structures
7. ____emia; excess blood starch
8. ___ology; the science of dosage
9. The large back teeth
10. _____sis; scientific investigation
11. _____morph; large
12. Roman 1003
13. Toward the mouth
18. Dental calculus
19. _____cology; science of drug uses and effects
24. _____oid; resembling jaundice
25. _____ Palsy; facial nerve paralysis
27. Highly active antiretroviral therapy (abbrev)
28. Chronic progressive external ophthalmoplegia (acronym)
29. Acute sensory axonal motor neuropathy (abbrev)
30. The hollow of the hand or foot
31. Roman 103
32. _____geny; development of an organism
33. _____osis; a bodily passage narrowing
34. _____sophy; system of beliefs
35. Monsters
37. _____phobia; fear of ghosts
38. Sensation of impending vomiting
43. _____rhagia; hemorrhage from a breast
44. _____ation; crying
45. _____ cranial nerve; glossopharyngeal
46. Temporary stop
47. Plants living in water
48. Walking manners
49. _____osis; degeneration of collagen fibers
50. Gangrenous inflammation of the mouth or genitalia
51. Adenosine deaminase acting on RNA (acronym)
52. _____algia; homesickness
53. Repose after exertion
56. ___ophobia; fear of disease
57. ___idic; pertaining to scales

10

Across

1. U.S. OB/GYN gp.
5. Shellac
10. Old
14. ____tropy; myocardial relaxation
15. Thin serous discharge from a wound
16. Spouse
17. Tooth alignment appliance used to manage prosthetic problems
20. Eastern equine encephalomyelitis (abbrev)
21. A spiral
22. ____ology; study of insects
23. A ripe ovum
25. Diffused matter in air
27. Toward the sacrum
29. Compulsive eating of nonfood substances
30. Organic mood syndrome (acronym)
33. ____ocyte; burr cell
34. ____mare; horrible dream
35. Consume
36. ____encephalon; forebrain
37. Psychoneurosis
38. ____geny; development of an organism
39. Brownish skin colour
40. Pertaining to the nose
41. ____oid; resembling a star
42. Adrenoleukodystrophy (abbrev.)
43. ____nal; everlasting
44. Arm bones
45. Forces sexual intercourse
47. Perspiration
48. Belief in traditional doctrines
50. ____dity; air dampness
51. ____ology; science of the development of ideas
54. Inflammation of intestine and liver
58. Cauda ____
59. Male ejaculatory fluid
60. ____tern; reservoir
61. ____uria; rapid urine excretion during fasting
62. ____ology; study of a cell's three-dimensional aspects
63. ____oid; star-shaped

Down

1. Plant derived juice used on skin
2. Effective disease treatment
3. Inflammation of bone and cartilage
4. Growth hormone-inhibiting hormone (acronym)
5. Resembling fat
6. Unpleasant to the smell or taste
7. ____uria; presence of bile in blood
8. Chief of Staff (abbrev)
9. ____iculation; joint
10. ____rrhea; abnormal stoppage of the menses
11. Inflammation of the stomach and intestines
12. ____tropic; directed against the cause
13. ____algia; pain in a ligament
18. Occurring every 8th day
19. ____itis; inflammation of the liver
24. Fetor ____; halitosis
25. A period of sleeplessness or wakefulness
26. Dull
27. Sagittal partitions dividing the nasal airways
28. Affecting the extremities
29. Hairy
31. Dura ____; outer brain and spinal cord membrane
32. ____form; cartwheel-patterned
34. Olfactory organs
37. The ultimate outcome
38. ____dysphoria; abnormal dislike of certain odors
40. ____algia; kidney pain
41. A posttreatment record review
44. Characterized by kindness
46. ____osis; incomplete development of the body
47. Above or beyond (prefix)
48. ____metry; size estimation of the unborn child
49. Anionic neutrophil-activating peptide (abbrev)
50. ____ralopia; day blindness
52. ____raction; act of diverting
53. ____ogen; female sex hormone
55. ____iferous; producing bone
56. ____erophonia; change of voice at puberty
57. Islet cell antibody (abbrev)

11

Across

1. The upper limb bend
6. Scratch trigger
10. ____esthesis; light sensitivity
14. A magnifying lens
15. Prefix meaning half
16. ____form; resembling a network
17. Increasing metabolic activity
20. The source of cocaine
21. Move swiftly on foot
22. Artery wall layers
23. Small skin outgrowths
25. Vessels
26. Single-celled organism (variable)
29. Unit of food energy (abbrev.)
30. ____pedic; clubfooted
34. A pouch
35. Atypical squamous cells of undetermined significance (acronym)
37. Skeleton parts
38. Between the metatarsals
41. ____genesis; asexual reproduction
42. Heat
43. ____flexia; lack of reflexes
44. ____tive; a demulcent remedy
45. ____ines; dogs
46. Possessing force
48. ____iculus; small elevation
50. Anti____; poison neutralizer
51. ____logy; linguistics (variable)
54. ____ital; of a finger
55. Tunica
59. Study of body divisions (2 words)
62. ____phobia; fear of heights
63. Inflammation of (suffix)
64. A diseased person
65. ____cephalon; betweenbrain, interbrain
66. ____oris; erectile female organ
67. ____humeral; shoulder joint

Down

1. ____tive; not essential
2. ____scelism; illness produced by brown recluse spider
3. ____inator; cheek muscle
4. Any medication containing opium
5. Damp
6. Antitr____; spasm that prevents closing the mouth
7. Puberty person
8. Certified Medical Transcriptionist (abbrev)
9. Referring to an opening
10. A muscle that turns a part downward
11. ____osis; sunstroke
12. Aural
13. Habitual spasmodic muscular movements
18. The acme of the sexual act
19. Bartholin glands (abbrev)
24. ____gnosis; inability to sense weight
25. Relating to a vessel
26. ____ism; absence of saliva
27. Skin disease of domestic animals
28. Occurring every 8th day
29. ____eous; of the skin
31. Looplike structures
32. Gain knowledge through experience
33. A small cluster of cells
36. Relating to the 1st part of the large bowel
37. ____itis; ear problems due to pressure
39. Urination
40. ____osis; sensation location recognition
45. Relating to clonus
47. Relating to a rooflike structure
49. ____dynia; earache
50. ____ole; heart relaxation phase
51. By degrees (abbrev.)
52. ____thin; emulsifying phospholipid
53. Monster
54. Roman 552
56. To exude moisture
57. Acute motor axonal neuropathy (abbrev)
58. ____genous; originating in cheese
60. Adult T-cell leukemia (abbrev)
61. ____esthesia; ability to sense pain

12

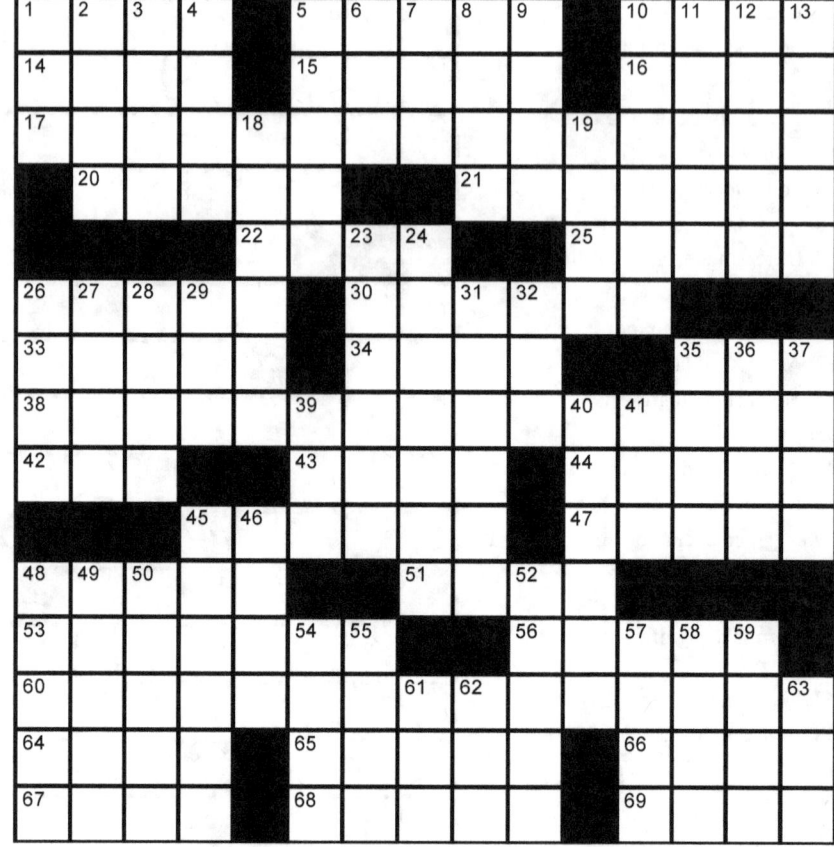

Across

1. A proton donor
5. Referring to the ankle
10. Superior aortic curve
14. Dimethyl sulfoxide (abbrev)
15. The soul or life
16. ____otomy; cutting operation in the vagina
17. Fear of a glare of light
20. Bone ridge
21. Nervelike
22. The body of a nerve cell
25. Mild
26. Taxonomic category between subfamily and genus
30. Congenital absence of one or more limbs
33. Warms
34. ala ____; outside flaring wall of each nostril
35. ___biosis; resuscitation
38. Enfolding of a segment of intestine within another
42. ____epinephrine; a vasoconstrictor
43. ____ology; study of disease
44. ____menia; occurrence of menstrual ulcers
45. Inability to speak
47. A point of origin
48. Fleshy lobe of the soft palate
51. ____culus; joint
53. Slackens
56. ____omosis; blood vessel coalescence
60. Within the cerebellum
64. The average
65. ____acoustic; of equilibrium and hearing
66. Prefix meaning thousand
67. Tumors (suffix)
68. ____philic; readily stained with osmic acid
69. Smallest unit of an element

Down

1. Adenosine 5-diphosphate (abbrev)
2. Community mental health center (abbrev)
3. ____rhea; maintenance of water equilibrium
4. Anti____; poison-stopping substance
5. Prefix meaning 'the same'
6. ___iitis; blood vessel inflammation
7. Roman 52
8. Acute motor axonal neuropathy (abbrev)
9. Forceful unconsentual sexual intercourse
10. Insatiable appetite
11. Automaton
12. Roman 153
13. Caputs
18. Evaluate
19. ____dity; air dampness
23. Performed by the hand
24. Absence of one or more mammary glands
26. Lean or slender
27. ____genic; originating in the kidney
28. ____ology; the science of medicine
29. British thermal unit (abbrev)
31. Scab formed after a burn
32. Fetal attitude or position
35. Angioimmunoblastic lymphadenopathy with dysproteinemia (abbrev)
36. ____ceptor; free nerve ending that detects pain
37. ____emia; absence of oxygen in arterial blood
39. A health resort
40. Norepine____; a neurotransmitter
41. An infusion or decoction
45. Fills with fear
46. ____tive; purgative
48. ____genous; of urinary origin
49. Poisonous secretion of an animal
50. Extreme
52. Restricted, prohibited, or forbidden
54. Enteric cytopathogenic swine orphan (abbrev)
55. Reduces a fracture
57. ____line; baselike
58. A long narrow opening
59. Prefix relating to the ankle bone
61. ___itis; nerve branch inflammation
62. ___ology; study of disease causes
63. The extent that a joint will move (abbrev.)

13

Across

1. ____phagia; ingestion of an excessive quantity of salts
5. ____sightedness; myopia
9. Roman 702
14. ____ism; coitus interruptus
15. Prefix meaning 'work'
16. Heat
17. ____algia; tooth pain
18. ____motor; related to movements caused by sound
19. Ascend
20. Relating to occiput and face
23. _____stenosis; constriction of the arteries
24. Relaxin (abbrev)
25. ____encephaly; occipital cranial defect
26. ____vert; withdrawn 'or' outgoing person
28. 'Dead on arrival' (abbrev)
31. _____ferous; yielding milk
34. ____pagus; twins joined at the occiput
35. Angioimmunoblastic lymphadenopathy with dysproteinemia (abbrev)
36. Relating to external ear and skull
39. Leglike part
40. Small mass of foreign cells
41. Walking manners
42. ___cup; diaphragmatic spasm
43. ____opia; night vision
44. ___algia; referred pain
45. ____phobia; fear of bees
46. Mold, yeast, mildew etc.
49. Relating to the umbilicus and intestine
54. A period in the course of a disease
55. ____licus; navel
56. French for AIDS
57. Pertaining to hair
58. ____osis; state of stupor

Down

1. ____phobia; fear of traveling
2. ____oic; echo-free
3. Incise with a sharp object
4. Inflammation of the innermost layer
5. _____ectomy; excision of the islet cells of the pancreas
6. ____genic; causing sexual arousal
7. ____genic; idiopathic
8. Upper surface of an anatomical structure
9. Roman 851
59. ____tia; denoting lack of force
60. _____phobia; fear of small skin parasites
61. Lateral attachment of inguinal ligament (abbrev)
62. ____ular; sphincteral muscle shape

10. A wine-cup
11. Clinical Laboratory Improvement Amendments (abbrev)
12. Infraorbitomeatal line (abbrev)
13. Institutional review board (abbrev)
21. Extreme and unreasoning anxiety and fear
22. _____escent; branching like a tree
26. ____osis; failure of ossification
27. ____urate; to urinate
28. Roman 503
29. Other licensed antifungal therapies (abbrev)
30. Normal everyday actions (abbrev)
31. ____rymal; relating to tears
32. ____form; ear-shaped

33. ____iate; cross-shaped
34. ____pexy; surgical fixation of ileum
35. Pain relieving drug
37. An ounce (Latin)
38. Active substance capable of producing an effect
43. ____cyte; a small
44. Artery wall layers
45. Newborn's health test score
46. _____cant; causing fever
47. _____ferous; Conveying urine
48. _____osis; hyperferremia
49. Aural
50. The cheek
51. ____tic; mentally ill person
52. Tumors (suffix)
53. ____inogenic; causing cancer
54. A health resort

14

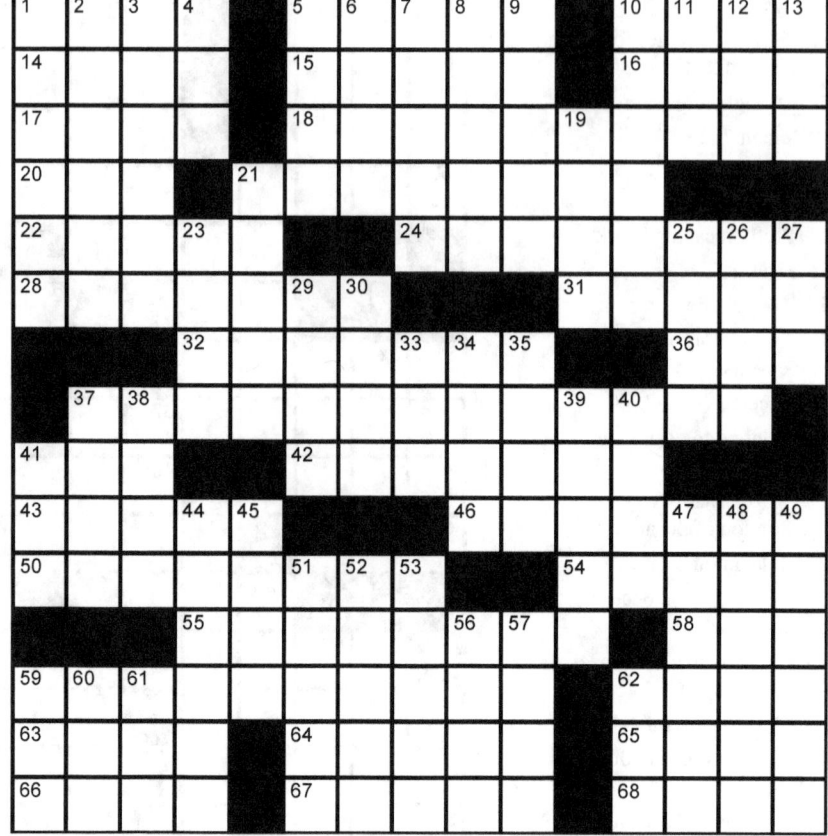

Across

1. Frequency of an event per unit of time
5. _____lary; microscopic blood vessel
10. Prefix meaning 'on all sides'
14. _____tive; not essential
15. _____cide; mite-destroying agent
16. _____uria; normal urination
17. _____tern; reservoir
18. Institution for the promotion of health
20. Electron beam tomography (abbrev)
21. Creaking, harsh-sounding
22. Period of rest for body and mind
24. Relating to the an organ's outer layer
28. Having a broad base of attachment
31. Small saclike gland dilatations
32. Craniometric point in the region of the sphenoid fontanelle
36. Isoelectric point (abbrev)
37. Pertaining to both mind and body
41. Counterimmunoelectrophoresis (abbrev)
42. Small bone
43. Roman 1062
46. Surprise suddenly
50. Abnormal overgrowth of the body
54. Blood fluid minus blood cells and clotting agents
55. Able to feel
58. Inosine 5-monophosphate (abbrev)
59. To encounter something personally
62. P-aminobenzoic acid (abbrev)
63. Mark left after healing
64. _____gnosia; denial of a neurological deficit
65. Atypical glandular cells of undetermined significance (acronym)
66. 16 fluid ounces (U.S.)
67. _____oid; shaped like a crown
68. ____itis; inflammation of a ligament

Down

1. A small hollow
2. Capable of nourishing
3. Male gonads
4. Electroconvulsive therapy (abbrev)
5. Protective plaster shell
6. _____ology; study of mites and ticks
7. Extreme and unreasoning anxiety and fear
8. _____malacia; softening of the iris
9. Metric unit of capacity
10. Referring to the main artery
11. A computerized diagnostic technique (abbrev)
12. British thermal unit (abbrev)
13. Unit of electric resistance
19. _____gonist; agonist's opposer
21. Expectorates
23. To catch sight of
25. Roman 103
26. _____dotal; based on case histories
27. Labium
29. _____myosarcoma; malignant tumor of the uterus muscle
30. The sum of all instincts for self-preservation
33. ___ation; masturbation
34. Acid___; abnormally high acidity
35. _____algia; night pain
37. Hairs
38. Prefix denoting 'six'
39. Osteo_____; bone tissue resorbing cell
40. _____ditary; transmissible from parent to offspring
41. Cystometrogram (abbrev)
44. To attach distally
45. A tubular passage
47. Process of sorting patients according to their need for care
48. The loin
49. A dusting powder
51. Relating to the inion
52. _____cephaly; narrowness of the head
53. Lesser
56. Enteric cytopathogenic swine orphan (abbrev)
57. Chemical element Ne
59. Mental telepathy (abbrev)
60. Roman 91
61. ___phobia; fear of everything
62. Soft material forming a cushion

15

Across

1. ___gnosia; denial of a neurological deficit
6. ___omy; body structure study
10. Elicits a tendon reflex
14. Unit of measure of frequency
15. ___facient; substance that warms
16. Enzyme-multiplied immunoassay technique (abbrev)
17. ___genic; denoting response to medical treatment
18. Active range of motion (abbrev)
19. A people
20. Brain part concerned with smell
23. ___algia; tooth pain
24. ___bian; female homosexual
25. ___lip; upper lip defect
28. ___oid; resembling death
31. ___urate; to ripen
34. ___virus; disease transmitted by rodents
36. Insect parasite that causes scabies
37. A single
38. Inflammation of stomach and intestines
42. ___erus; jaundice
43. Roman 1007
44. ___osis; failure of ossification
45. Oral Hygiene Index (abbrev)
46. Resembling hair
49. Contralateral routing of signal (acronym)
50. Desquamative interstitial pneumonia (abbrev)
51. ___ceptor; free nerve ending that detects pain
53. Inability to recognize or orient part of one's own body
60. ___ation; micturation
61. ___atrial node; pacemaker
62. ___osis; liver disorder
64. ___phobia; fear of strangers
65. ___grity; soundness of structure
66. ___pelvis; twisted pelvis
67. ___ology; medical science
68. Puberty person
69. ___ology; study of dreams

Down

1. Apnea-hypopnea index (abbrev)
2. ___sightedness; myopia
3. ___uria; normal urination
4. Creaking or harsh-sounding
5. Oxidizing agent; O3
6. ___osis; thickening of the stratum spinosum
7. ___osis; state of stupor
8. Plant derived juice used on skin
9. A pattern or mold
10. A malformed fetus
11. ___gam; cavity filler
12. Prefix meaning 'one trillionth'
13. ___osis; a bodily passage narrowing
21. ___eric; of the small intestine
22. ___delphus; unequal conjoined twins
25. ___therapy; religious treatment of the sick
26. ___noid; weblike
27. ___form; ropelike
29. ___rrhexis; rupture of the amniotic membrane
30. Louse egg
31. Muscle contraction neuron
32. ___coria; asymmetric pupils
33. Examinations
35. Axilla
39. To lay eggs (insects)
40. ___oid; resembling a coil or roll
41. The act of cutting
47. Groin
48. Deoxynivalenol (abbrev)
50. One that gives
52. Prefix meaning 'modified by heat'
53. ___lytic; increasing the destructive power of a lysin
54. Chief nitrogenous endproduct of protein metabolism
55. A shade of a color
56. Nore___phrine; a neurotransmitter
57. ___brachium; forearm
58. ___versible; permanent
59. ___culus; joint
63. ___cus; axillae odor

Across

1. ____chondria; energy producing organelles
5. Obstructive sleep apnea-hypopnea syndrome (abbrev)
10. ___emia; intestinal autointoxication
14. ___lysis; destruction by cold
15. Extreme anxiety and fear
16. ___dynia; foot pain
17. Cartilage oligomeric matrix protein (acronym)
18. Lying within the meshes of a network
20. Moving in the same direction at the same time (2 words)
22. Con___ion; impregnation prevention
23. ___ology; metaphysical study of the nature of existence
24. ___ferous; yielding milk
25. An artificial joint
32. ___gnosis; lack of sensory recognition of a limb
33. ___mentition; reproduction by germination
34. ___pose; fatty
37. Unit of apparent loudness
38. ___algia; intestinal pain
39. Antineutrophil cytoplasmic antibodies (abbrev)
40. Extraocular muscles (abbrev)
41. Body structure with a specific function
42. ___oic; echo-free
43. Collapse of lung tissue
45. Any open skin lesions
49. Decay
50. Craniometric point on sagittal suture near lamboid suture
53. Referring to the thigh
57. Traveling of a disease from one part to another
59. ___chism; a taste for suffering
60. Lateral attachment of inguinal ligament (abbrev)
61. Deficient in active properties
62. Isopropylthiogalactoside (acronym)
63. Bed covering for administering oxygen
64. Overcomes difficulties
65. Wax

Down

1. Roman 1201
2. Fe
3. ___anal; resonant
4. Rarely used term for ovary
5. ___otic; behind the ear
6. Of sound mind
7. ___acid; acid buffering substance
8. ___ellous; resembling fine hairs
9. Mark left after healing
10. A figure-eight bandage
11. ___tomy; excision of the large intestine
12. Adjust to different conditions
13. ___pelvis; twisted pelvis
19. Untrue
21. ___gonist; agonist's opposer
25. The back of the neck
26. Sound repetition
27. Active range of motion (abbrev)
28. Difference between the limits of a variable
29. Relating to the number 8
30. Exhibition of questionable behavior
31. ___uption; a breaking through
34. ___thesia; lack of sensation
35. Roman 701
36. Infection-associated hemophagocytic syndrome (abbrev)
38. Estrogen replacement therapy (abbrev)
39. Related to the structure of the body
41. Something that provides refuge
42. Smallest unit of an element
44. Bone ridges
45. ___algia; body pain
46. Excessively overweight
47. ___itis; inflammation of the optomeninx
48. ___osis; degeneration of collagen fibers
51. Aural
52. Prefix meaning 'one billionth'
53. One of the 5 elements
54. Forceful unconsentual sexual intercourse
55. ___oid; star-shaped
56. ___phasia; inability to speak
58. ___sis; toxic condition

17

Across

1. Wing-like process
4. ___onic; having equal tension
8. A figure-eight bandage
13. Hairs
15. ___uria; rapid urine excretion during fasting
16. To imitate or simulate
17. ___ism; coitus interruptus
18. Diffuse unilateral subacute neuroretinitis (acronym)
19. Beginning
20. Sweat
23. Cotton plugs
24. A stoppage of flow
28. ___ectomy; removal of the ileum
29. ___exia; state of ill health
31. Certified Medical Assistant (abbrev)
32. ___ogenic; promoting tear secretion
35. ___itis; inflammation of the testis
36. Disease-spreading rodent
37. Study of ecologic influences on human health
41. ___iatry; study and treatment of speech disorders
42. Olfactory organ
43. Dura ___; outer brain and spinal cord membrane
44. ___chanter; bony elevation
45. Bed covering for administering oxygen
46. ___gut; suture material
47. Female sibling
49. Knee cap
53. Person in their eighties
56. Active substance capable of producing an effect
59. Blood donors deposit place
60. ___vert; both extrovert and introvert
61. Suffix meaning 'pain'
62. Feminine suffix
63. ___myosarcoma; malignant tumor of the uterus muscle
64. Inner or central
65. Time the earth takes to revolve around the sun
66. ___ sequitur; 'it does not follow' (Latin)

Down

1. ___osis; cell suicide
2. Narrow ridge or streak
3. Fear aroused by awareness of danger
4. Element/mineral used in the synthesis of thyroid hormones
5. Spiked bone projections
6. Bones
7. A shade of a color
8. 'Unstriated' or 'involuntary' muscle type
9. Auricle
10. Intramuscular stimulation (abbrev)
11. Abbrev. for counterimmunoelectrophoresis
12. Activated clotting time (abbrev)
14. Inhale
21. Any growth protruding from a mucous membrane
22. ___algia; sciatica
25. ___itis; inflammation of the testes sac
26. Vivid mental picture
27. ___iasis; male hypersexuality
29. Bone ridge
30. Critical stage of a disease
32. Short for shoulder muscles
33. ___cide; mite-destroying agent
34. ___trum; initial breast fluid
35. ___toid; tooth-shaped
38. Deficient in active properties
39. Tumors (suffix)
40. On the side
45. Relating to a rooflike structure
46. Painful mouth sore
48. Amyo___; muscle tone defect
49. Prefix denoting 5
50. The external opening of a space
51. ___nasal; relating to the lips and nose
52. Negatively charged ion
54. To follow commands
55. To close an ion channel
56. ___noid; gland-like
57. Gynecology (abbrev)
58. ___eric; of the small intestine

Across

1. ___thin; emulsifying phospholipid
5. Rate of change of position with time
10. ___sthesia; pain sense
14. ___eurosis; sheet-like tendon
15. ___meter; speed measuring device
16. Heat injury
17. Short for sugar or starch
18. Group of eight
19. ___emia; intestinal autointoxication
20. Pertaining to the kinesthetic sense
23. ___algia; nose pain
24. A command or direction
25. ___tion; the process of knowing
28. Hollow area of bone
31. ___oid; morphine-like
32. ___motor; relating to voluntary movements
35. End result of coagulation
39. Study of body divisions (2 wds)
42. ___nestic; assisting the memory
43. Wears away
44. Intermittent acute porphyria (acronym)
45. A stupid person
47. Rigid
49. Causing death
52. ___ cell; any precursor cell
54. Agent that causes vomiting and purging
60. ___men; earwax
61. ___ology; study of dreams
62. ___olic; growth enhancing steroid
64. ___rant; deviating
65. Examines with a sensing device
66. Tubular bone shape
67. Treat with a light beam device
68. The trunk
69. ___sis; absence of germs

Down

1. Any whitish milklike liquid
2. Expiratory positive airway pressure (acronym)
3. ___ugator; wrinkle-producing muscle
4. As if from birth
5. ___form; cartwheel-patterned
6. ___itis; inflammation of the pacinian corpuscles
7. ____genous; originating outside the organism
8. Enterohemorrhagic Escherichia coli (acronym)
9. Anti___; poison-stopping substance
10. A condensed summary of a scientific article
11. Clear
12. Severe or serious
13. _____algia; intestinal pain
21. Prefix meaning 'to like'
22. ___ology; the science of dosage
25. ____coid; scapular process
26. Not obstructed
27. Prefix signifying one billion
28. Villain
29. Toward the mouth
30. A unit of perceived loudness
33. ____tia; denoting lack of force
34. Prefix referring to pressure
36. Lumbus
37. Tumors (suffix)
38. To assign a character or category
40. Lacking complete growth
41. ___oid; resembling a star
46. ___phonia; impaired speech
48. Emergency Medical Treatment and Labor Act (acronym)
49. Relating to bodily waste
50. Single-celled organism (variable)
51. ___ major; arm adductor
52. Anterior legs
53. Prefix referring to the ankle
55. ___algia; rib pain
56. ___neus; elbow muscle
57. Lacrimal gland secretion
58. ___emia; excess fibrin in the blood
59. Walking stick
63. Acronym for bone Gla protein

19

Across

1. Cauda
5. Illuminating device
9. ___grade; moving backward
14. Place of refuge and safety
15. Chief end product of nitrogen metabolism
16. Thin serous discharge from a wound
17. Effective renal plasma flow (acronym)
18. ___osis; state of stupor
19. ___therapy; cancer treatment
20. Pertaining to balance and hearing
23. Roman 3
24. Corticotropin-releasing hormone (acronym)
25. A covering
28. ___itis; inflammation of the testes sac
30. Belonging to the female
32. Brownish skin colour
33. Situated between
36. Structures of threadlike appearance
37. Tonic muscular spasm preventing mouth closing
39. Roman 701
41. Excessive hunger
42. ___cum; prefix meaning 'around'
43. ___itude; a sense of weariness
44. Not general or systemic
48. Colour produced by the shortest visible spectrum waves
50. A soft food for babies or invalids
52. ___didymus; single body conjoined twins
53. Referring to the midbrain
57. Small saclike gland dilatations
59. Chinese philosophical masculine principle
60. ___iorrhea; excessive
61. ___genic; causing sexual arousal
62. Clinical Laboratory Improvement Amendments (acronym)
63. ___roid; resembling a dream
64. Enzyme released by the kidney
65. Lacrimal gland secretion
66. ___phobia; fear of the dawn

Down

1. Proposition submitted for a doctorate
2. Referring to the main heart artery
3. To weaken in quality
4. The spleen side
5. Resembling the moon in shape
6. ___noid; weblike
7. ___genesis; reproduction by segmentation
8. Postanesthesia care unit (acronym)
9. A fissure
10. Prefix meaning 'spiny'
11. Inflammation of a tendon sheath
12. The extent that a joint will move (abbrev.)
13. ___facial; relating to the mouth and face
21. Group of eight
22. Internal stimulus creating imbalance
26. Unit of food energy (abbrev)
27. ___biosis; resuscitation
29. ___present; everywhere
30. Injures
31. ___tropic; directed against the cause
34. To expand or swell
35. Inflammation of (suffix)
36. ___cellular; spindle-celled
37. Lateral part of the spine of the scapula
38. ___osis; loss of the eyelashes
39. Roman 605
40. Roman 102
43. A pathologic change in the tissues
45. Large intestine (prefix)
46. Highest points
47. ___rrhea; excessive post-childbirth vaginal discharge
49. ___form; lens-shaped
50. ___phobia; fear of poverty
51. Newborn's health test score
54. ___algia; night pain
55. ___facient; substance that warms
56. Plant derived juice used on skin
57. ___osis; production of gas in the tissues
58. ___master; testis-suspending muscle

20

Across

1. ___phobia; fear of touch
6. Hollows
10. Adrenal androgen-stimulating hormone (acronym)
14. Dull pains
15. ___itis; inflammation of the female gonad
16. Hooked anatomical processes
17. One who prepares and dispenses drugs
19. Crust of a superficial sore
20. A covering structure or roof
21. Roman 502
22. ___otomy; cutting operation in the vagina
23. Finger or toe
25. Resembling the moon in shape
26. Roman 1205
30. A living, sentient organism
32. Chief artery supplying the head
35. Capable of being cut or divided
39. Ring-shaped
40. Instrument for removing tartar from teeth
41. The constitution of tissues
43. A surface covering
44. Imperfect or incomplete development
46. ___phobia; fear of the dawn
47. A lung
50. Inner; central
53. ___osia; drinking of urine
54. Intraventricular block (acronym)
55. ___emia; blood poisoning
60. Seizure made with the teeth
61. The functional elements of an organ
63. ___tia; denoting lack of force
64. Walking unit
65. A rounded swelling
66. Tender
67. ___phalanx; a toe bone
68. ___osis; failure of ossification

Down

1. ___ometer; touch-sensitivity measuring instrument
2. Dull pain
3. ___ology; the subject of eating
4. A specified period of time
5. Acronym for otospondylomegaepiphysial dysplasia
6. ___cyx; tailbone
7. Antibiotin
8. Inflammation of the ductus deferens
9. ___culus; joint
10. To listen to bodily sounds
11. Elbow
12. A stairlike structure
13. ___nation; winter sleep
18. ___lingus; sexual stimulation of the anus
24. Glutamate decarboxylase (acronym)
25. Shellac
26. Med. school applicant's test (abbrev)
27. Walking stick
28. A junction or crossing
29. A unit of electrical power
31. ___morph; large
33. ___meric; relating to the same part
34. ___versible; permanent
36. ___psoas; hip flexor
37. Focusing device
38. Prefix meaning 'work'
42. To raise up
43. ___gut; suture material
45. Rooted and ingrained in one's nature
47. Anteroinferior portion of the hip bone
48. ___genous; of urinary origin
49. Metric unit of capacity
51. Asparagine (abbrev)
52. Ate___sis; collapse of lung tissue
54. Inhibitory postsynaptic potential (acronym)
56. Unit of apparent loudness
57. ___genous; originating in cheese
58. Most inferior of several similar structures
59. Protective plaster shell
62. Prefix meaning 'upon' or 'above'

21

Across

1. HIV/AIDS reporting system (acronym)
5. ___itis; inflammation of the heart
9. Toward the median plane of the body
14. ___dotal; based on case histories
15. Winglike structures
16. Inwardly
17. Second stage in insect development
18. Incapable of normal locomotion
19. ___itis; inflammation of adipose tissue
20. Transfer of genetic code information from one nucleic acid to another
23. Roman 3
24. Mini stroke (abbrev)
25. Having many branches
28. ___algia; heart pain
30. ___algia; leg pain
32. ___physis; a line of union
33. Suffering from Hansen disease
36. Congenital or sympathetic
37. Inflammation of the middle layer of the aorta
39. Hamulus
41. Gives enjoyment to
42. Adeno-associated virus (acronym)
43. Shades or tints
44. Immune stimulating complexes (acronym)
48. ___choline; neurotransmitter
50. ___ology; the study of fungi
52. ___oid; morphine-like
53. Referring to the midbrain
57. Active substance capable of producing an effect
59. Consumes
60. ___sightedness; myopia
61. A faculty of perceiving a stimulus
62. ___form; shaped like a leather bottle
63. ___genous; originating outside the organism
64. ___algia; intestinal pain
65. Unit of acoustic impedance
66. ___osis; a bodily passage narrowing

Down

1. Relating to the sense of touch
2. Absence of urine formation
3. Restore damaged tissues
4. Survey by traversing with a sensing device
5. ___ferol; vitamin D
6. Acronym for as low as reasonably achievable
7. Nerve branches
8. Away from the surface
9. Nearer the dental arch center line
10. ___ology; study of insects
11. Abnormal narrowing of a duct
12. Abdominal aortic aneurysm (acronym)
13. Dichlorodiphenyltrichloroethane (acronym)
21. Inflammation of the sebaceous glands of the eyelids
22. Perforation
26. ___arthrodia; fibrous joint
27. Acronym for emergency medical dispatcher
29. Deep lamellar endothelial keratoplasty (acronym)
30. Open skin lesions
31. ___neous; of the skin
34. A pimple-like formation
35. Behavior pattern individuals present to others
36. To salute with the lips
37. The act of motion
38. ___opsia; migraine aura
39. Hepatitis-associated antigen (acronym)
40. Oculoauriculovertebral dysplasia (acronym)
43. ___ectomy; surgical removal of the uterus
45. ___asia; distention of the large intestine
46. Any medication containing opium
47. One-millionth of a meter
49. Rigid
50. Process of measuring (suffix)
51. ___iform; Y-shaped
54. ___algia; nerve pain
55. ___menia; menstruation
56. ___thesia; lack of sensation
57. Suffix meaning 'enzyme'
58. ___eric; nonproprietary

22

Across

1. As low as reasonably achievable (acronym)
6. ___icle; collarbone
10. ___omy; body structure study
14. Walking sticks
15. A pigmented fleshy skin growth
16. ___algia; nerve pain
17. Osteo___; bone tissue resorbing cell
18. Roman 26
19. ___ology; study of hearing
20. Relating to umbilicus and intestine
23. ___present; everywhere
24. ___momania; morbid compulsion to count
25. Steam baths
28. ___cardia; incomplete heart development
31. A division or portion
32. Anal injection of fluid
33. Cumulative trauma disorders (acronym)
36. ___osis; hereditary multiple exostoses
40. ___emia; sulfur in the blood
41. Bone ridge
42. Roman 541
43. ___malacia; softening of the lens
44. Pertaining to a lack of oxygen
46. ___rhea; normal uterine discharge
49. Unit of apparent loudness
50. Agent that causes vomiting and purging
56. Specific sites
57. ___roid; resembling a dream
58. A stupid person
60. ___phia; a wasting away
61. ___eolus; ankle process
62. ___ acid; protein part
63. Inert gaseous atmospheric element
64. Plant derived juice used on skin
65. Light beam device

Down

1. Anodal closure contraction (abbrev)
2. ___chezia; emotional discharge gained by uttering indecent words
3. ___nestic; assisting the memory
4. Any action evoked by a stimulus
5. An inflammatory lung disease
6. Roman 941
7. ___scelism; clinical illness produced by the brown recluse spider
8. ___olus; oxygen exchange pocket
9. A return blood vessel
10. ___genic; producing no gas
11. ___tis; inflammation of a nerve
12. A posttreatment record review
13. ___ology; study of hair
21. Autonomic nervous system (abbrev)
22. Referring to the ankle
25. Macula
26. Adrenal androgen-stimulating hormone (acronym)
27. ___caria; hives
28. ___gnosia; denial of a neurological deficit
29. Bed covering for administering oxygen
30. Emergency medical dispatcher (acronym)
32. Enterohemorrhagic Escherichia coli (acronym)
33. Roman 920
34. ___pedic; clubfooted
35. Dacarbazine (abbrev)
37. ___dermia; yellow skin discoloration
38. ___vat; a type of cloth bandage
39. Tumor of the teeth forming tissues
43. A large dose of liquid medicine
44. U.S. hospital gp.
45. Typical; usual
46. ___cholia; a mental depression
47. To give expression to feeling
48. ___phobia; fear of dying
49. 'A lover or admirer' (suffix)
51. Extreme unresponsive brain state
52. ___eptic; nervous system stimulant
53. ___phase; final stage of mitosis
54. Rainbow-like eye part
55. Retinal photoreceptor for acute color vision
59. ___epinephrine; a vasoconstrictor

23

Across

1. ___phia; a wasting away
5. To join together
10. Diethylenetriamine pentaacetic acid (abbrev)
14. Relating to urine
15. An eminence or elevation
16. ___itis; tenosynovitis
17. Sensitive aesthetic perception
18. Kidney waste product
19. ___dynia; labor pains
20. Between the teeth
23. ___pathia; seasickness
24. ___phagy; the eating of excrement
25. To close an ion channel
26. Autonomic nervous system (abbrev)
27. ___algia; pain in a limb
28. Bronchoalveolar lavage (abbrev)
31. Expectorated matter
33. Capable of moving
36. Gangrenous inflammation of the mouth or genitalia
37. Excessive sodium excretion in the urine
40. ___iate; cross-shaped
42. The forcible striking of one body against another
43. Toward the back part
46. Familial erythrophagocytic lymphohistiocytosis (abbrev)
47. Antidiuretic hormone (abbrev)
50. Insulin-like activity (abbrev)
51. ___morphosis; change of form
54. ___geny; absence or defect of a bodily part
56. ___gut; suture material
57. A mucous discharge from the anus
60. My___; nearsightedness
62. To express grief or sorrow
63. Time earth takes to revolve around the sun
64. ___rhea; maintenance of water equilibrium
65. Epitympanic recess
66. Proximal upper limb parts
67. ___algia; tooth pain
68. ___rrhagia; hemorrhage from the nipple
69. Olfactory organ

Down

1. 'Extreme withdrawal' (mental disorder)
2. Sleeplike state of altered consciousness
3. Pertaining to a fissure
4. Group of eight
5. ___al; inferior
6. Monster
7. Growing older
8. Prefix denoting five
9. Gives medical aid to
10. Diphtheria
11. The death instinct
12. 'Through the anus' (2 words)
13. Hearing sounds that are not there
21. Automaton
22. ___idic; pertaining to scales
29. Auditory brainstem response (abbrev)
30. Roman 53
32. One of the components of a whole
33. ___ocyte; large red blood cell
34. ___bus; loin
35. Effective renal plasma flow (abbrev)
37. Involuntary nodding
38. Experimental allergic encephalitis (abbrev)
39. ___osis; pathological tissue hardening
40. Ring-shaped
41. Return of a disease
44. Adenosine monophosphate (abbrev)
45. ___itis; inflammation of the skin
47. ___sclerosis; arterial wall deposit accumulation
48. Sleep images
49. Having a noisy voice
52. Dens
53. Sharp or severe
55. ___esthesia; inability to perceive cold
58. ___ogy; series of three
59. ___genesis; origin and growth of a neoplasm
61. ___iculation; joint

24

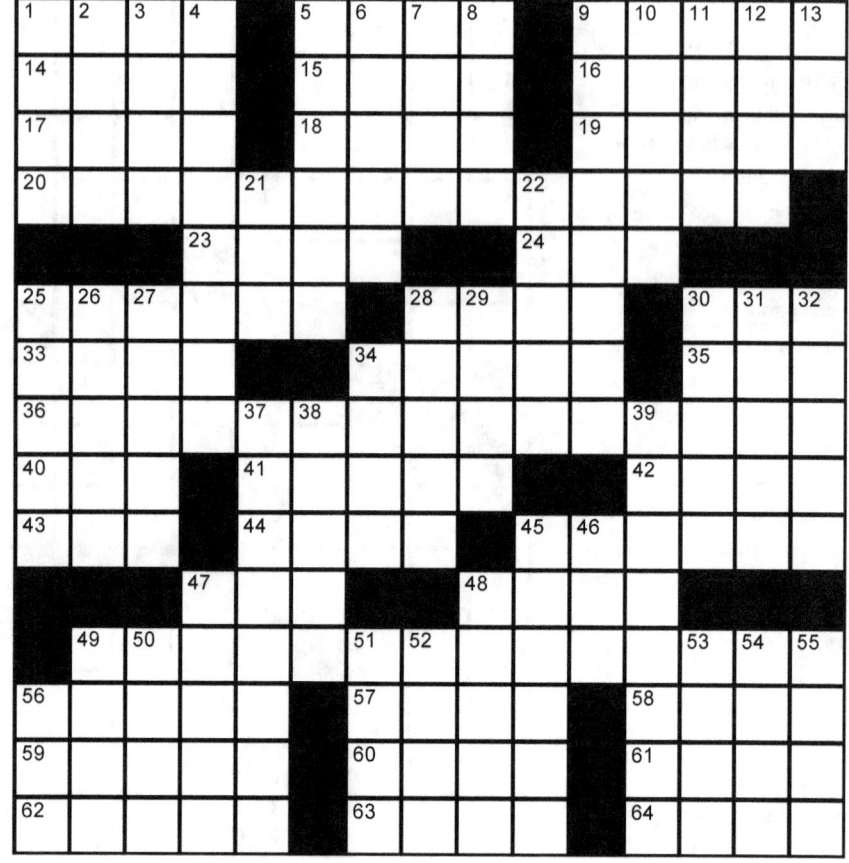

Across
1. Violent anger
5. A quantity of matter
9. Relating to the wall of any cavity
14. ___thesia; lack of sensation
15. Hooked anatomical processes
16. ___algia; female gonad pain
17. ___ilage; joint covering
18. A sitting surface
19. Space within a tubelike structure
20. Defective unilateral development of the limbs
23. ___mania; abnormal liking for music
24. Chimpanzee coryza agent (abbrev)
25. A sawing movement in massage
28. Postanesthesia care unit (abbrev)
30. External hordeolum
33. Sensitive aesthetic perception
34. ___lary; microscopic blood vessel
35. To elicit a tendon reflex
36. Involving both the arterioles and the veins
40. ___profen; analgesic and anti-inflammatory agent
41. Surface borders
42. ___culus; joint
43. ___ophobia; fear of disease
44. ___blast; nucleus of the fertilized oocyte
45. ___oid; resembling smallpox
47. Basle Nomina Anatomica (abbrev)
48. ___egenation; interbreeding of different race
49. Fear of neglect of duty
56. Body structure with a specific function
57. Walking stick
58. ___ology; anatomy of the soft parts of the body
59. Pertaining to sound
60. ___rhea; liquid feces
61. ___onic; having equal tension
62. Severe pain
63. Adult respiratory distress syndrome (abbrev.)
64. Breaks moral laws

Down
1. ___itis; inflammation of the vertebral column
2. ___robic; without oxygen
3. A pathogenic microorganism
4. A rough calculation
5. Skeletal
6. ___derma; looseness and atrophy of the skin
7. Mark left after healing
8. ___toxin; a food poison
9. Smallest unit of a substance
10. Fleshy lobe of the soft palate
11. Nerve branches
12. Part of a surface
13. ___itis; inflammation of gastric cellular tissue
21. Brain scan (abbrev)
22. Roman 1204
25. To dye
26. ___hydrate; sugar or starch
27. A sudden attack
28. Prefix meaning 'old'
29. ___taxis; slight hemorrhage
30. ___form; cartwheel-patterned
31. Prefix meaning 'the same'
32. ___iform; Y-shaped
34. ___ition; the process of knowing
37. The briefest unit of experience
38. A standard of perfection
39. A state of stupor
45. Venomous snakes
46. Asymmetric septal hypertrophy (abbrev)
47. Cranial cavity mass
48. A unicellular organism
49. Progesterone (abbrev)
50. ___genic; idiopathic
51. International Classification of Diseases (abbrev)
52. Two objects considered together because of similarity
53. ___lar; referring to a foundation
54. Fe
55. Performs
56. Obstructive sleep apnea (abbrev)

25

Across

1. ___phobia; fear of religious or sacred objects
6. ___cide; mite-destroying agent
11. AIDS dementia complex (abbrev)
14. Beneath
15. ___cephalon; endbrain
16. Prefix meaning 'in front of' or 'favoring'
17. Proximal to phalanges
19. ___comenia; occurrence of menstrual ulcers
20. ___phobia; fear of spiders
21. Neither artificial or pathologic
23. Habitual spasmodic muscular movement
24. Abnormal dryness of the conjunctiva
25. Grows older
28. Egg shaped
32. Foot (prefix)
33. Cross-reacting material (abbrev)
34. Nostril
36. Unexpected infant death (abbrev.)
39. Enteroinvasive Escherichia coli (abbrev)
41. Severe pain or extreme suffering
42. ___esis; suppression of a discharge
43. Insulin-dependent diabetes mellitus (abbrev)
44. Space within a tubelike structure
45. ___acus; hip flexor
46. ___form; grape-shaped
48. ___ology; anatomy of the soft parts of the body
49. Chief or principal
50. An appliance for fixation of displaced or movable parts
53. ___nism; coitus interruptus
55. Wine-cups
57. An external application
61. Wing-like process
62. Resection of an intestinal segment
64. Short for arm adductor
65. ___rrhea; drooling
66. Spiral in form
67. Had food
68. Any wasting of the body
69. ___genic; causing sexual arousal

Down

1. ___nosis; a people disease that is spread to other animals
2. ___tia; denoting lack of force
3. Ethylenediaminetetraacetic acid (abbrev)
4. Responds to a stimulus
5. ___algia; pain in the testes
6. ___phia; a wasting away
7. Congenital erythropoietic porphyria (abbrev)
8. ___ine; an amino acid
9. To slacken
10. The arch of the foot
11. Extreme sexual desire
12. Sleep image
13. ___genosis; connectve tissue disease
18. Relating to the elbow
22. ___esthesia; the normal urge to urinate
25. Angiotensin-converting enzyme inhibitors (abbrev)
26. A chart with horizontal and perpendicular lines for plotting curves
27. To remove bone marrow
29. 10th cranial nerve
30. An agreeable odor
31. Internal layer of protective material
35. Sudden
37. Roman 651
38. Anterior border of tibia
40. Roman 907
47. Prohibited sexual intercourse between relatives
49. Anything that occupies space and has mass
50. A stairlike structure
51. ___itis; inflammation of the roof of the mouth
52. Any anatomic bandlike structure
54. An indentation
56. Pierce with a pointed instrument
57. The sum of all instincts for self-preservation
58. ___gram; three-dimensional image
59. Enzyme-multiplied immunoassay technique (abbrev)
60. ___cyte; a mucous tissue cell
63. ___ment; constituent part

26

Across
1. ___meter; pupillometer
5. High-frequency oscillatory ventilation (abbrev)
9. ___osis; loss of the eyelashes
14. Egg shaped
15. ___morph; large
16. Irregularly notched
17. Seeking or attracted to light
19. ___ mortis; death state
20. Final letter of the Greek alphabet
21. Surgical instrument for cutting bone
23. Used to express disgust
25. ___scope; lung capacity measuring device
26. System of treating disease by body manipulation
32. Openings or foramina
33. Plural of genus
34. ___sis; toxic condition
37. Euthan___; mercy killing
38. ___algia; ankle pain
39. Breakout of pimples
40. Foot (prefix)
41. Piri___; external hip rotator
44. ___algia; breast pain
45. Morbid fear of pleasure
47. Squamous
49. ___titis; inflamation of the main artery
50. Sharp-pointed
54. ___ectopia; floating spleen
58. ___encephalia; absence of the cerebellum
59. Final stage of mitosis or meiosis
61. A salt of uric acid
62. Repose after exertion
63. ___tent; closed
64. Biological units of heredity
65. ___mania; compulsive shopping
66. ___exia; absence of fever

Down
1. Prefix meaning 'large intestine'
2. Female reproductive cell
3. A people
4. Urin deficiency
5. Human monocytotropic ehrlichiosis (abbrev)
6. ___metry; size estimation of the unborn child
7. Obstructive sleep apnea syndrome (abbrev)
8. A unit of electromotive force
9. Partial blindness
10. Referring to iris inflammation
11. ___rhea; excessive talking
12. ___phagia; swallowing food without thorough mastication
13. ___ditary; transmissible from parent to offspring
18. ___phagia; compulsive eating of ice
22. ___ogen; female sex hormone
24. Hypothalamic-pituitary-gonadal (abbrev)
26. Continuous positive airway pressure (abbrev)
27. A section of open-ended flexible tubing
28. ___ectomy; surgical removal of part of the iris
29. ___grade; moving backward
30. ___esis; recollection
31. ___ma; abdominal tumor
34. Crust of a superficial sore
35. ___form; xiphoid
36. Prefix signifying one quadrillion
39. The quality of being shapeless
41. Cats
42. ___acusis; painful sensitivity to noise
43. A health resort
45. Wrist bone with a 'hook'
46. ___ital; health care institution
47. Numerical evaluation of achievement
48. ___eous; of the skin
50. Acute necrotizing ulcerative gingivitis (abbrev)
51. ___phia; a wasting away
52. Puberty person
53. Ethical legal and social implications (acronym)
55. Illuminating device
56. To catch sight of
57. ___sightedness; myopia
60. ___dynia; earache

27

Across

1. ___mentition; reproduction by germination
6. Antibody-dependent cell-mediated cytotoxicity (abbrev)
10. ___egenation; interbreeding of different race
14. Nostrils
15. ___algia; hand pain
16. Prefix meaning 'eight'
17. Occurrence of menstrual symptoms without bleeding
20. Discharge from the ear
21. ___osis; cell suicide
22. Extraocular muscles (acronym)
23. ___iorrhea; excessive post-childbirth vaginal discharge
25. Grows older
28. Abnormal fear of flashes of light
34. A toothlike structure
35. ___ferous; yielding milk
36. Decay
37. ___eric; of the small intestine
38. ___mastia; abnormally large breasts
39. Adverse drug reaction (abbrev)
40. ___ mater; deep membrane covering the brain and spinal cord
41. ___tis; inflammation of the urinary bladder
42. Roman 1003
43. Innervated bone area
46. ___ordination; ataxia
47. ___genic; originating in the kidney
48. A neck flexor (abbrev)
50. A stupid person
53. Relating to weakness
58. Incision of the sclera and iris
61. A measure of duration
62. An impulse
63. Mispronounces the sibilants S and Z
64. Obstructive sleep apnea syndrome (abbrev)
65. Lost blood
66. Group of eight

Down

1. ___neus; elbow muscle
2. ___ilage; joint covering
3. ___lysis; destruction by cold
4. To exclude unconsciously from the conscious mind
5. ___genic; estrus-producing
6. Critical stage of a disease
7. Dehydroepiandrosterone (abbrev)
8. Cervical intraepithelial neoplasia (abbrev)
9. Cathode ray oscilloscope (abbrev)
10. ___logy; science of the forms and structure of organisms
11. ___roid; denoting a thin purulent discharge
12. A walking unit
13. Tunica
18. Electric resistance units
19. ___centesis; lumbar puncture
23. ___ation; crying
24. ___kinetic; pertaining to eye movement
25. Lard
26. Obeso___; causing obesity
27. Inner
29. ___lysis; dissolution of elastic fibers
30. ___genesis; milk production
31. Cranial cavity mass
32. Relating to iodine
33. ___megaly; enlargement of an atrium
38. An individual muscle unit
41. ___cyte; red blood cell with serrated edges
42. Having the nature of imitating
44. Wears away
45. ___ogen; female sex hormone
49. ___genetic; producing bile
50. ___chondria; energy producing organelles
51. Fetor ___; halitosis
52. A cleft or crack
53. ___sthesia; pain sense
54. Sperm
55. ___algia; homesickness
56. ___tus; the motor element of an instinct
57. An enclosed fluid-filled sac
59. Prefix meaning 'below'
60. Crown-rump length (acronym)

28

Across

1. ___dacism; disarticulation of the letter L
5. A unicellular organism
10. Brainstem auditory evoked potential (abbrev)
14. Antineutrophil cytoplasmic antibodies (abbrev)
15. ___cyte; red blood cell with serrated edges
16. ___lytic; increasing the destructive power
17. Binaural alternate loudness balance test (abbrev)
18. Exists
19. ___osis; a bodily passage narrowing
20. Renewal of life and strength
23. Kidney waste product
24. Human granulocytotropic ehrlichiosis (abbrev)
25. VD
27. ___ety; any equal part
28. ___cephalon; most recently evolved brain part
32. Hard, white tooth covering
34. Any pencil-shaped structure
36. ___formis; external hip rotator
37. Skin sensation of prickling or creeping
40. Like a wing
42. Pertaining to the iris
43. ___cision; foreskin removal
46. A looplike structure
47. ___endix; vermiform process
50. ___lateral; affecting only one side
51. ___bian; female homosexual
53. A pathologic startle syndrome
55. Treatment of disease in the aged
60. ___blast; an independent cell
61. A spot or blemish
62. C2
63. Prefix meaning 'oil'
64. ___itis; blood vessel wall swelling
65. 'Eyelid' (prefix)
66. Protective plaster shell
67. Gain knowledge through experience
68. A luminous or colored circle

Down

1. Rim
2. ___genic; producing no gas
3. Roman 1157
4. ___skis; newborn foot reflex
5. Roman 1151
6. Open reduction and internal fixation (abbrev)
7. Moles and birthmarks
8. ___oic; echo-free
9. The measured quantity of a drug
10. ___lar; referring to a foundation
11. Awareness of one's own body odor
12. ___itis; inflammation of intestinal peritoneal covering
13. Metallic bone implant
21. ___icular; relating to a heart chamber
22. ___algia; tendon pain
26. Roman 551
29. Oculus
30. Ethical legal and social implications (acronym)
31. ___ceutical; functional food
33. ___otomy; incision into an apical structure
34. ___ology; anatomy of the body's soft parts
35. Anterior border of tibia
37. Organ or cavity walls
38. Ehlers-Danlos syndrome (abbrev)
39. ___mesis; vomiting of saliva
40. ___ology; study of therapeutic needle use
41. A small tonguelike structure
44. ___trichous; having curly hair
45. Referring to the mind or chin
47. Inability to coordinate movements
48. ___itis; inflammation of the optic disk
49. ___genic; caused by normal body activity
52. To look fixedly
54. ___noid; weblike
56. Lowermost attaching structure
57. Prefix meaning 'eight'
58. ___ology; study of mammals
59. ___iated; structure protruded through an opening
60. Anodal opening contraction (abbrev)

29

Across

1. ___phagy; the eating of excrement
6. Sudden involuntary muscle contraction
11. ___atitis; liver inflammation
14. Occurring on the 9th day
15. ___gamy; sexual promiscuousness
16. Intermediolateral (abbrev)
17. Epitympanic recess
18. Pertaining to the distal small intestine
19. A health resort
20. Surgical reconstruction of the renal pelvis
22. ___algia; tendon pain
23. Sodium chloride
24. Having little height
26. Parasitic insects
30. Congenital absence of one or more limbs
31. Dull pains
32. Study of body structures
35. Dirt
36. ___algia; toothache
37. ___esis; suppression of a discharge
40. Kidney
42. Larynx sound
43. A disease
45. ___itis; inflammation of an organ-enclosing sheet
46. Large back tooth
47. Residue remaining after percolation of a drug
49. 7th letter of the Greek alphabet
50. Referring to faint sounds produced by the ear
57. ___algia; referred pain
58. Thin walls dividing two cavities
59. Surgical incision (suffix)
60. ___encephaly; occipital cranial defect
61. Between (prefix)
62. ___ erythematosus; chronic inflammatory disease
63. Computed tomography angiography (abbrev)
64. ___form; cartwheel-patterned
65. ___osis; bone mass within a bone

Down

1. A short sharp sound
2. ___loid; cup-shaped
3. ___brachium; forearm
4. Cauda
5. Condition marked by neoplasm development
6. Overflow
7. ___itis; inflammation of the roof of the mouth
8. ___thesia; lack of sensation
9. With no delay
10. ___phobia; fear of infection
11. Disintegration of tissue
12. ___polesis; penetration of one cell by another
13. Sole of the foot
21. ___phobia; fear of everything
25. ___algia; pain in one eye
26. A body vessel
27. Prefix meaning 'habitat'
28. Nasalized speech
29. Passage of dark-colored tarry stools
30. ___enuate; to diminish
32. Adverse drug reaction (abbrev)
33. ___tropics; brain enhancers
34. Autonomic nervous system (abbrev)
36. Unit of electric resistance
38. Critical care unit (abbrev)
39. ___comenia; occurrence of menstrual ulcers
41. Heartburn
42. A space in the cytoplasm of a cell
43. An agent that induces vomitting
44. Possessing force
45. Cathode ray oscilloscope (abbrev)
47. Dura ___; outer brain and spinal cord membrane
48. ___cide; mite-destroying agent
51. Bed covering for administering oxygen
52. ___kinetic; pertaining to eye movement
53. Render unconscious by cerebral trauma
54. ___phobia; fear of certain places
55. Most inferior of several similar structures
56. An enclosed fluid-filled sac

30

Across

1. ___ology; study of disease causes
4. A vivid mental picture
9. An agreeable odor
14. ___bian; female homosexual
15. Roman 702
16. Buttocks
17. The self
18. ___ment; feces
19. ___algia; toothache
20. Ulceration at the umbilicus
23. A type of cell division during gamete production
24. A water jet for internal cleansing
27. ___nestic; assisting the memory
28. ___motor; stimulating the sweat glands
31. Dirt
32. Exercise-induced bronchospasm (abbrev)
35. Circular band surrounding an opening
37. Soft material forming a cushion
38. The presence of only one digit on a limb
41. Chronic idiopathic urticaria (abbrev)
43. With no delay
44. ___nism; coitus interruptus
45. Alternate binaural loudness balance (abbrev)
47. ___itis; tenosynovitis
49. Time the earth takes to revolve around the sun
53. Reciprocal
55. Hold back for future use
58. Insect-eating
61. Prefix meaning 'head'
63. Light beam device
64. Roman 551
65. Heat
66. Speak one`s opinion without fear or hesitation
67. Suffix referring to the female
68. ___virus; disease transmitted by rodents
69. Examinations
70. To reduce a fracture

Down

1. Oil tumor
2. A covering structure or roof
3. Equality of vision in both eyes
4. Mental conceptions
5. Roman 1141
6. A means of admittance
7. A female youth
8. Enteroinvasive Escherichia coli (abbrev)
9. ___gnosia; denial of a neurological deficit
10. Lateral forearm bone
11. The examination of the ear
12. Adult males
13. Aspartate aminotransferase (abbrev)
21. ___stasis; state of equilibrium
22. ___lith; dental calculus
25. ___tus; an opening
26. ___erly; old
29. A salt of uric acid
30. Disseminated intravascular coagulation (abbrev)
33. ___anity; severe mental illness
34. ___-feeding; breastfeeding substitute
36. Abbreviation for gynecology
38. ___ sclerosis; neurological disease
39. Disordered action of heart (acronym)
40. Panniculus
41. Complementary and alternative medicine (abbrev)
42. ___profen; analgesic and anti-inflammatory agent
46. Abnormal prominence of the great toe
48. A significant life-changing event
50. Wears away
51. To tear away a body part
52. Stand firm against
54. ___phobia; fear of thunderstorms
56. Specific occurrence
57. Any open skin lesions
59. End result of coagulation
60. Synthetic material used as a suture
61. Chimpanzee coryza agent (abbrev)
62. Antigen-antibody reaction (abbrev)

31

Across

1. Round flat anatomical structure (variable)
5. Enteric cytopathogenic swine orphan (abbrev)
9. Sound repetition
13. Prefix meaning 'seven'
14. Bronchiolitis obliterans with organizing pneumonia (abbrev)
15. The mentum
16. ___birth; birth material expelled
17. Hooked anatomical processes
18. Central part of a structure
19. Enlargement of the heart
21. Ethical legal and social implications (abbrev)
22. Stannum
23. ___algia; earache of nerve origin
25. Resembling the elbow
30. Estrogen replacement therapy (abbrev)
31. ___tropics; brain enhancers
32. Roman 800
34. ___oid; pulley-shaped
38. Fear of odors
42. Mental lethargy
43. ___utism; excessive bodily hair
44. ___oid; resembling a coil
45. Doctor of Dental Medicine (abbrev)
47. Tendency toward spontaneous coagulation of the blood
50. Temporal, frontal, parietal and sphenoid junction
54. Adult male
55. ___gram; three-dimensional image
56. Muscle cell plasma membrane
62. Rainbow-like eye part
63. Part of a surface
64. ___osis; blindness without apparent eye change
65. ___tropy; myocardial relaxation
66. Bent (like a knee)
67. Perceive flavour in the mouth
68. Obstructive sleep apnea syndrome (abbrev)
69. Suffix meaning 'condition'
70. ___itis; inflammation of a bone

Down

1. ___cation; discharge of feces
2. Isopropylthiogalactoside (abbrev)
3. ___lysis; fat emulsion in the digestive process
4. ___osis; widely spread cancer
5. A tissue resembling ivory
6. ___uction; transmission
7. ___pathic; manifesting antisocial traits
8. Medication containing opium
9. ___piesis; pressure exerted outward from within
10. ___sterol; a steroid
11. ___tism; excessive bodily hair
12. ___ology; study of dreams
13. ___string; posterior knee tendon
20. Positive electrode
24. ___uria; normal urination
25. ___aly; deviation from normal
26. ___mania; hypochondriacism
27. ___ology; study of feces
28. Interstitial cell-stimulating hormone (abbrev)
29. Roman 603
33. A thickening of the skin on the toes
35. Small triangular membrane formed at the caudal angle of the rhomboid fossa
36. Roman 103
37. ___zone; drinking water sterilizer
39. Production and excretion of sweat
40. Nerve branches
41. ___phagia; swallowing food without thorough mastication
46. The measured quantity of a drug
48. ___plegia; paralysis of the soft palate
49. Anal injections of fluid
50. Prefix meaning 'to like'
51. A swelling or bulging projection
52. Enzyme-linked immunosorbent assay (abbrev)
53. Nostrils
57. ___capsule; capsule of the kidney
58. ___algia; burning pain
59. ___algia; breast pain
60. Person who does not speak
61. ___flexia; lack of reflexes

32

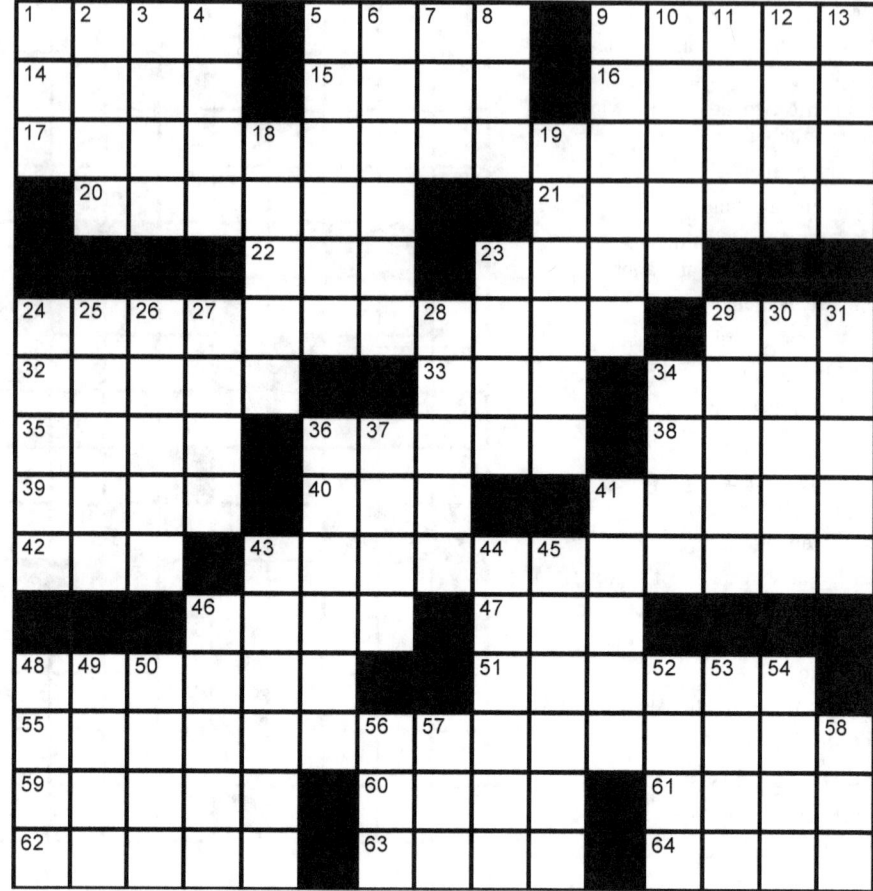

Across

1. ___aphobia; fear of public places
5. A return blood vessel
9. ___osis; blindness without apparent eye change
14. Cheek
15. ___tus; the motor element of an instinct
16. Prefix meaning 'four'
17. Study of diseases of the nails
20. Breath out
21. Hard white tooth covering
22. ___osis; production of gas in the tissues
23. Ache
24. Saclike outpouchings of the colonic wall
29. U.S. dental grp.
32. Stupid person
33. ___flexia; lack of reflexes
34. ___algia; leg pain
35. Reduces a fracture
36. An internal layer of protective material
38. Certified Registered Nurse Practitioner (abbrev)
39. ___tid; neck artery
40. ___biosis; resuscitation
41. Belief in traditional doctrines
42. ___genous; of the same origin
43. Incomplete development of the heart
46. ___rant; deviating
47. ___nation; micturation
48. ___rhagia; hemorrhage from a breast
51. Sore
55. Inflammation of the intestine and liver
59. A stairlike structure
60. Most inferior of several similar structures
61. ___atrial node; pacemaker
62. A ripe ovum
63. Frequency that an event occurs per unit of time
64. ___ition; the process of knowing

Down

1. Gone by
2. Biological unit of heredity
3. A claw or nail
4. ___itis; inflammation of the vertebral column
5. Colour produced by the shortest waves of the visible spectrum
6. ___polesis; penetration of one cell by another
7. Isopropyl alcohol (abbrev)
8. Devoid of anything extraneous
9. Lack of muscle tone
10. ___cholia; a mental depression
11. Smallest unit of an element
12. An impulse
13. Unit of acoustic impedance
18. Highly active antiretroviral therapy (abbrev)
19. One who cures
23. Unadulterated
24. Rounded flat plates
25. Mental conceptions
26. In ___; within a test tube
27. ___phobia; fear of the dawn
28. A narrow passage
29. Sharp or pungent
30. ___stry; study of teeth
31. 1st letter of the Greek alphabet
34. Mark left after healing
36. ___deviation; displacement to one side
37. ___tia; denoting lack of force
41. Syncope
43. Directed away from the mouth
44. The amount produced by an entity during a specified time
45. A slight linear depression
46. ___osis; incomplete development of the body
48. ___morph; large strong body type
49. ___neus; elbow muscle
50. With no delay
52. Round flat anatomical structure (variable)
53. ___tropic; directed against the cause
54. Circular band surrounding an opening
56. ___cus; axillary hair
57. Swelling (suffix)
58. ___burn; erythema solare

33

Across

1. The supporting structure of nervous tissue
5. ___esthesia; phantom limb pain
10. Suffering from disease
14. ___anal; resonant
15. Small saclike gland dilatations
16. ___tis; inflammation of the large intestine
17. Superiormost masticatory muscle
19. ___toid; tooth-shaped
20. Abbreviation for acetaminophen
21. Speak one`s opinion without fear or hesitation
22. ___cide; mite-destroying agent
25. Excretion of uric acid in the sweat
29. The extremities of any axis
30. Glove and condom material
31. Roman 1101
32. ___esis; an eruption or rash
34. Congenital erythropoietic porphyria (abbrev)
35. Yellow-colored
42. ___ety; any equal part
43. ___ment; percussive massage movement
44. ___encephalon; middle brain
47. Relating to the cheek
49. Enzyme released by the kidney
50. Greek philosopher and scientist
52. Bone ridge
53. ___tosis; prolapse of the large intestine
54. ___osis; direct nuclear division
56. ___itis; inflammation in the womb
57. Within or enclosed by the dura mater
63. Narrow elevation of a bone
64. Aches
65. ___capsule; capsule of the kidney
66. Performs
67. ___omosis; blood vessel coalescence
68. Enzyme-multiplied immunoassay technique (abbrev)

Down

1. Glucose tolerance test (abbrev)
2. An alkaline percolate from wood ashes
3. ___unogen; antigen
4. Obvious or evident
5. Near, beside, beyond (prefix)
6. ___algia; shoulder blade pain
7. ___oid; resembling a coil or roll
8. Prefix meaning 'one'
9. ___ability; impaired function
10. ___philia; voyeurism
11. Poisoning by iodine
12. Relating to clonus
13. ___ology; the study of body movements
18. ___otic; behind the ear
21. Orexin (abbrev)
22. Tip of a structure
23. The hip joint
24. ___ine; an amino acid
26. Spinal
27. A tubular passage
28. A bodily distribution area
33. ___stasis; state of equilibrium
36. ___agious; communicable
37. Emaciating
38. An opening in a structure
39. A sound of distinct frequency
40. Inflammation of (suffix)
41. ___rum; middle point of a body
44. Spot or blotch on the skin
45. Lustful
46. Producing no detectable signs or symptoms
47. Guanosine triphosphate (abbrev)
48. Gains knowledge through experience
51. Any open skin lesions
55. ___algia; breast pain
57. Isopropyl alcohol (abbrev)
58. ___ism; dwarfishness
59. Mini stroke (abbrev)
60. Dream state (abbrev)
61. ___lingus; sexual stimulation of the anus
62. ___mus; acidity or alkalinity indicator

34

Across

1. ___kinesis; movement in the body tissue
6. A complete bend in a vessel forming a circular ring
10. ___egenation; interbreeding of different race
14. Mental conceptions
15. ___rhea; maintenance of water equilibrium
16. ___line; having a pH greater than 7.0
17. Respond to a stimulus
18. ___chondria; energy producing organelles
19. Spleen
20. Slow involuntary movements of the hands
23. Hearing organ
24. Anti___; poison-stopping substance
25. U.S. doctors gp.
28. ___myosarcoma; malignant tumor of the uterus muscle
31. Suppuration
35. ___duct; seminal duct or uterine tube
37. A particular condition of functioning
39. ___algia; pain in the sole of the foot
40. Ovarian pain or neuralgia
43. Relaxes
44. ___mania; compulsive shopping
45. ___opia; night vision
46. A lung disorder
48. Bones
50. ___matomania; preoccupation with specific names or words
51. The smallest of a litter
53. ___algia; referred pain
55. Involuntary backward gait
61. Other licensed antifungal therapies (abbrev)
62. ___form; resembling a network
63. Absence of autonomic breathing
65. ___bel; loudness measurement unit
66. ___ation; micturation
67. Prefix meaning 'four'
68. Foot digits
69. ___rate; soften by wetting
70. A defect in structure or function

Down

1. ___cus; axillary hair
2. Mental conception
3. A sitting surface
4. A spot or blemish
5. Relating to bone
6. ___sis; abnormal hunger
7. Acid___; abnormally high acidity
8. A ripe ovum
9. ___algia; facial pain
10. Rounded ankle joint process
11. ___psoas; hip flexor
12. A deviation from a symmetric pattern
13. ___ines; dogs
21. ___phobia; fear of involuntarily shaking
22. A tampon
25. ___phobia; fear of public places
26. Changes position
27. ___omosis; blood vessel coalescence
29. ___therapy; treatment with iodine
30. ___meter; pain measuring instrument
32. ___blast; myoblast
33. The external occipital protuberance
34. ___acoustic; of equilibrium and hearing
36. Inflammation of a joint
38. Suffix meaning 'condition'
41. Antitr___; spasm that prevents closing the mouth
42. ___phobia; fear of returning home
47. A nearly closed cavity
49. To add air to
52. ___peutic; curative
54. A person with Hansen disease
55. Prefix meaning 'oil'
56. Rate of movement
57. Aural
58. Nore____phrine; a neurotransmitter
59. ___insic; of internal origin
60. ___genesis; the formation of gas
61. Optical Doppler tomography (abbrev)
64. Antigen-antibody reaction (abbrev)

35

Across

1. Galvanic skin response (abbrev)
4. ___mentition; reproduction by germination
9. A proton donor
13. ___tive; not essential
15. Pertaining to wild, untamed animal
16. Openings or foramina
17. Opposition
19. A division or portion
20. ___dynia; pain in the uterus
21. Relating to speech or to the voice
23. Volatile or distilled liquids
26. Adult male
27. Relating to fatty heart
33. An illicit drug
37. Any weblike tissue
38. ___algia; heart pain
39. Specific occurrence
41. Endometrial intraepithelial neoplasia (abbrev)
42. Monsters
43. Near, adjoining (prefix)
44. Roman 107
46. Abbreviation for eye, ear, nose and throat
47. Muscular weakness
50. British thermal unit (abbrev)
51. Involving accurate and vivid recall
56. Absence of a spleen
61. ___cardia; incomplete heart development
62. Near beside beyond (prefix)
63. An agent that relieves retention of urine
66. ___taxis; slight hemorrhage
67. ___oid; shaped like a crown
68. ___iate; cross-shaped
69. Prefix meaning 'after'
70. ___form; cartwheel-patterned
71. ___ous; lacking muscular tissue

Down

1. Pathogenic microorganisms
2. State of partial unconsciousness
3. ___form; rope-shaped
4. ___osa; foot-and-mouth disease
5. Carcinoembryonic antigen (abbrev)
6. Certified Registered Nurse Practitioner (abbrev)
7. ___itis; inflammation of the vertebral column
8. Oil tumor
9. A structure attached to the body
10. Tunica
11. ___gate; to wash out
12. Round flat anatomical structure (variable)
14. ___hosis; liver disorder
18. Dirt
22. ___lepsy; paroxysmal sleep
24. Female breast (slang)
25. Vocal expression of thoughts
28. Oval eminence on medulla oblongata
29. Relating to dogs
30. ___versible; permanent
31. ___algia; gland pain
32. ___tern; reservoir
33. ___ vu; repetitive feeling
34. Female reproductive cell
35. Surgical fixation (suffix)
36. Cell nucleolus
40. Perceive flavour in the mouth
45. Roman 3
48. Artery wall layers
49. Adenosine deaminase acting on RNA (abbrev)
52. Enterotoxigenic Escherichia coli (abbrev)
53. Prefix meaning 'four'
54. The broad, flaring portion of the hip bone
55. ___geal; of the tailbone
56. Abbreviation for acetaminophen
57. ___naceous; soapy
58. ___encephalon; forebrain
59. ___onic; having equal tension
60. ___phobia; fear of heights
64. ___mone; bodily secretion
65. Prefix meaning 'one'

36

Across

1. Roman 1201
5. Expiratory positive airway pressure (abbrev)
9. ___duct; seminal duct or uterine tube
13. ___ine; an amino acid
14. ___capsule; capsule of the kidney
15. ___oia; sluggish mental activity
16. ___ose; milk sugar
17. Smell
18. Rigid and elevated
19. Excessive erotic interest
22. A small mass of foreign cells
23. ___gut; suture material
24. Rainbow-like eye parts
28. Denoting a parasite that infects the same host throughout its entire life
32. Prefix referring to 'tears'
33. ___osis; losing one's hair
35. ___dontia; absence of teeth
36. Between the neuromeres
40. Life time
41. Spherical bodies
42. ___ence; inability to copulate
43. Prefix meaning 'brain'
46. ___therapy; phototherapy
47. ___ulus; collection of cells
48. ___ocyte; large erythrocyte
50. Study of joint diseases
58. Nostril
59. A tubular passage
60. Winglike structures
61. ___ acid; protein part
62. Chicken embryo lethal orphan (virus)(abbrev)
63. ___menia; menstruation
64. ___motor; moving the hair
65. Euthan___; mercy killing
66. ___nal; everlasting

Down

1. Cheek
2. Gonorrhea (slang)
3. ___exia; state of ill health
4. ___insic; of internal origin
5. Wears away
6. Of the foot
7. ___osis; failure of ossification
8. ___formis; external hip rotator
9. Of a convoluted or ring shape
10. Not obstructed
11. ___ceptor; free nerve ending that detects pain
12. ___gonist; agonist's opposer
15. ___uria; blood in the urine
20. ___ology; study of dreams
21. ___dynia; eye pain
24. ___ crest; pelvic ridge
25. The difference between the limits of a variable
26. ___oid; resembling jaundice
27. Digital rectal examination (abbrev)
28. Ventilates
29. Extensor _____ radialis; wrist extensor
30. The external occipital protuberance
31. Prefix meaning 'modified by heat'
33. ___melia; congenital deformity of the limbs
34. Prefix meaning 'below'
37. ___cyte; healthy red blood cell
38. ___phallus; abnormally small penis
39. Emergency Medical Technician (abbrev)
44. ___cyte; burr cell
45. ___pathy; disease of a bursa
46. ___cyte; a colorless cell
48. Spouses
49. ___osis; incomplete body development
50. Anionic neutrophil-activating peptide (abbrev)
51. Nerve branches
52. ___ogy; series of three
53. Compulsive eating of nonfood substances
54. ___rated; torn
55. Other licensed antifungal therapies (abbrev)
56. To close an ion channel
57. Earth's revolve time around the sun

37

Across

1. Atypical glandular cells of undetermined significance (acronym)
5. A stairlike structure
10. A portion
14. Prefix referring to pressure
15. Artery wall layer
16. ___nal; everlasting
17. Aural
18. ___esis; recollection
19. A network or plexus
20. Excessive love of knowledge
23. Angiotensin-converting enzyme inhibitors (abbrev)
24. A sharp end or apex
25. Squamous
28. Thin specimen for examination
31. With, together (prefix)
32. Relating to light
35. ___eptic; nervous system stimulant
39. Study of diseases of the nails
42. Prefix meaning 'over a distance'
43. ___otropic; referring to weather-affected diseases
44. Chief of Staff (abbrev)
45. ___cephaly; narrowness of the head
47. ___practor; bone-setter
49. To spread or turn out
52. Dull pain
54. Morbid fondness for taking drugs
60. ___rated; torn
61. Substantia _____; midbrain part
62. Roman 1190
64. Ethyleneglycotetraacetic acid (abbrev)
65. A defect in structure or function
66. Mental conception
67. Inert gaseous element in the atmosphere
68. Bone ridge
69. ___pharynx; superior portion of the pharynx

Down

1. Symbol for blood group systems
2. To close an ion channel
3. ___osia; drinking of urine
4. Pertaining to living in a community
5. A condition
6. ___form; wedge-shaped
7. ___nestic; assisting the memory
8. ___sis; excessive hunger
9. American College of Nuclear Physicians (abbrev)
10. Around the mouth
11. ___osis; incomplete development of the body
12. ___itis; inflammation of the optomeninx
13. Give medical aid to
21. ___oid; cup-shaped
22. Hypothalamic-pituitary-adrenal (abbrev)
25. ___opia; night vision
26. Retinal photoreceptor for acute color vision
27. ___emia; excess blood starch
28. ___acoustic; of equilibrium and hearing
29. Insect parasite that causes scabies
30. Sound repetition
33. Place of refuge and safety
34. Not obstructed
36. ___ceptor; a receptor for pain
37. ___aphobia; fear of public places
38. Dissolution (prefix)
40. ___ section; baby removal procedure
41. ___algia; pain in the testes
46. ___panic; resonant
48. ___thophobia; fear of worms
49. ___ectopia; floating spleen
50. Eats or destroys (suffix)
51. ___genesis; milk production
52. ___opia; absence of the face
53. An information graph
55. ___dotal; based on case histories
56. ___hosis; liver disorder
57. Monster
58. International Classification of Diseases (abbrev)
59. Imaginary lines passing through the body's center
63. Conscious alert oriented (abbrev)

38

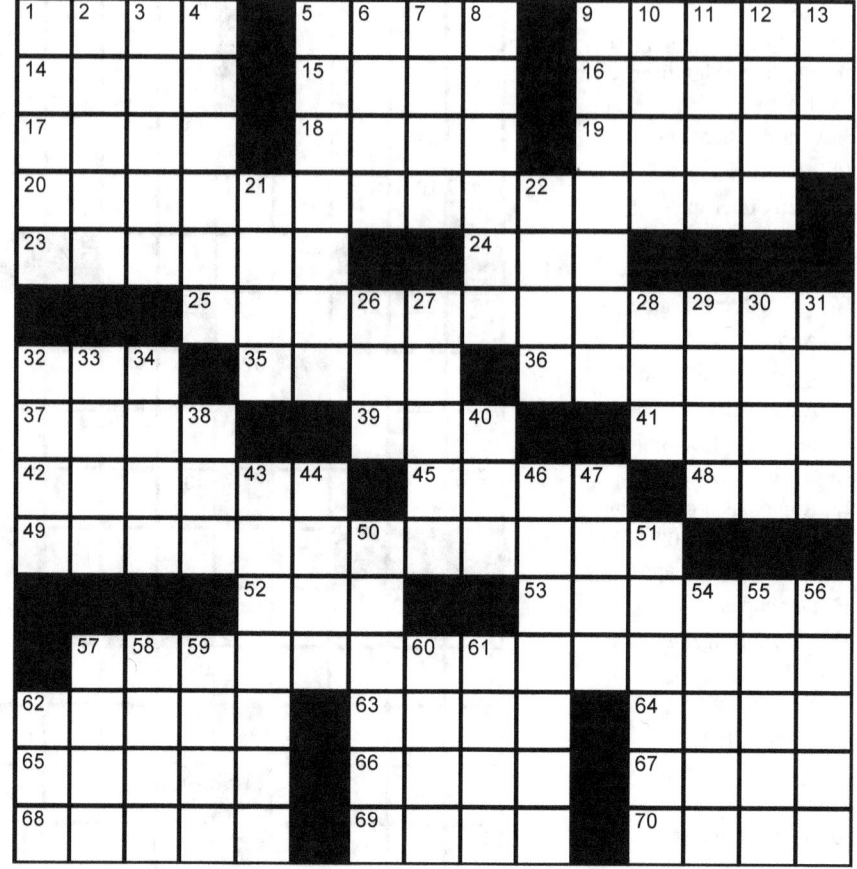

Across

1. Acute sensory axonal motor neuropathy (abbrev)
5. ___phthisis; emaciation from lack of nourishment
9. ___ation; gonad removal
14. Plural of nodus
15. ___osia; drinking of urine
16. The brain and spinal cord
17. Spoken
18. ___agious; communicable
19. A line
20. Posterior, medial hamstring muscle
23. The collagen of bone
24. ___date; heart-shaped
25. Not united into one bone (hyph.)
32. Caseous Lymphadenitis (abbrev)
35. ___anal; resonant
36. Simple eyes of insects
37. Nore___phrine; a neurotransmitter
39. Obstructive sleep apnea (abbrev)
41. To mispronounce the sibilants S and Z
42. Greek word for 'breath'
45. Idiopathic hypertrophic subaortic stenosis (abbrev)
48. Petroleum
49. Widely dispersed
52. Brain and spinal cord system (abbrev)
53. ___phobia; fear of being scratched
57. Relating to the ischium and perineum
62. ___eology; study of remains of past peoples
63. To breathe rapidly and shallowly
64. ___cans; becoming white
65. Cranial cavity mass
66. ___grity; soundness of structure
67. Roman 1054
68. ___grade; moving backward
69. ___aphobia; fear of public places
70. ___itis; bone inflammation

Down

1. ___gnosia; denial of a neurological deficit
2. Any open skin lesions
3. ___ apple; laryngeal prominence
4. Social and cultural surroundings
5. The state of being luminous
6. Fe
7. The seat of consciousness in the brain
8. The science of light and vision
9. Relating to heat
10. C2
11. ___atrial node; pacemaker
12. Foot digits
13. Carrier of genetic information (abbrev)
21. A shade of a color
22. ___mania; belief that one is suffering from a specific disease.
26. ___dynia; shoulder pain
27. Glycoprotein portion of a photopigment
28. Familial erythrophagocytic lymphohistiocytosis (abbrev)
29. ___psoas; hip flexor
30. Ethical legal and social implications (abbrev)
31. ___opia; double vision
32. Calcium pyrophosphate deposition disease (abbrev)
33. ___ment; medicament rubbed into the skin
34. ___thesia; lack of sensation
38. Endoscopic ultrasound (abbrev)
40. U.S. hospital gp.
43. ___phobia; fear of machinery
44. ___otic; fetus-surrounding fluid
46. Primer
47. Prefix meaning 'half'
50. Equality of vision in both eyes
51. Prefix meaning 'force'
54. Basic units of living things
55. An addiction
56. Oval eminence on medulla oblongata
57. ___versible; permanent
58. ___emia; intestinal autointoxication
59. ___algia; hand pain
60. A sudden
61. ___blast; a cell nucleolus
62. Auditory brainstem response (abbrev)

39

Across

1. A healing substance
5. Acrocephalosyndactyly (abbrev)
9. Suffix meaning 'measuring instrument'
14. A mental conception
15. Protective cover on the dorsal distal phalanges
16. Irregularly notched
17. ___rum; middle of body
18. ___iform; wedge-shaped
19. A noxious or poisonous substance
20. Narrowing of the intestinal lumen
23. A substance that is injurious to health
24. A soft food for infants
25. ___cardia; enlargement of the heart
28. Vitamin B3
33. ___archy; a system of things ranked one above the other
37. Medial forearm bone
39. ___dynia; eye pain
40. The production of sensation
43. Epitympanic recess
44. Female reproductive cell
45. ___onic; having equal tension
46. Pertaining to the lateral side of the palm
48. Lateral attachment of inguinal ligament (abbrev)
50. ___form; grape-shaped
52. A specimen of tissue collected for analysis
57. Referring to the heart and blood vessels
62. An abnormally elated mental state
63. ___lity; body function weakness
64. A standard
65. Specific occurrence
66. ___pexy; surgical fixation of ileum
67. Smallest unit of an element
68. A measuring device
69. ___ivore; flesh eating mammal
70. ___mania; abnormal talkativeness

Down

1. Elbow flexor
2. ___dynia; pain in a gland
3. ___form; lens-shaped
4. Spouses
5. Elbow muscle
6. ___algia; burning pain
7. 16 fluid ounces (U.S.)
8. State of partial unconsciousness
9. Craniometric point midway between the frontal eminences
10. The sum of all instincts for self-preservation
11. ___phobia; fear of being poisoned
12. Suffix meaning 'condition'
13. Kidney
21. The extent that a joint will move (abbrev)
22. ___ism; dwarfishness
26. ___blast; early neural cell
27. Acronym for analysis of variance
29. Angiotensin-converting enzyme inhibitors (abbrev)
30. Con___ion; brain injury
31. ___psoas; hip flexor
32. ___algia; homesickness
33. Warmth
34. ___mus; narrow passage between two parts
35. Feminine suffix
36. ___algia; nose pain
38. Atypical glandular cells of undetermined significance (acronym)
41. Tailless
42. A discharge
47. Roman 56
49. A pouch
51. Relating to iodine
53. Relating to the wall of any cavity
54. ___mania; a delusion of having great wealth
55. ___nosis; understanding of speech
56. ___phobia; fear of solitude
57. Hollows
58. ___rysm; blood vessel dilation
59. Circular band surrounding an opening
60. Veil-like structures
61. ___rant; deviating from normal
62. ___algia; very severe pain

40

Across

1. Clinical Laboratory Assistant (abbrev)
4. Elicits a tendon reflex
8. In a direction toward the inion
13. ____ment; bone-connecting tissue
15. A standard
16. The nape of the neck
17. ___olic; growth enhancing steroid
18. Spoken
19. Give medical aid to
20. Superficial three layers of transversospinal muscles
23. In front of the ear
24. Vomiting
28. An infusion or decoction
29. Part of a surface
31. Certified Medical Assistant (abbrev)
32. ___ulum; small head of a bone
35. ___dotal; based on case histories
36. Disease-spreading rodent
37. Study of nail diseases
41. Lower limb between the knee and the ankle
42. The measured quantity of a drug
43. Dura ___; outer brain and spinal cord membrane
44. Tumor (suffix)
45. Prefix meaning 'after'
46. Short for an arm adductor
47. The male fertilizing element of flowering plants
49. Knee cap
53. Person in their eighties
56. Head
59. ___aneus; heel bone
60. ___vert; both extrovert and introvert
61. To tantalize
62. A measure of duration
63. ___myosarcoma; malignant tumor of the uterus muscle
64. ___al; situated near the kidney
65. ___omy; body structure study
66. ___ism; dwarfishness

Down

1. A holding device
2. An internal layer of protective material
3. ___genesis; asexual reproduction
4. Abnormal deviation of the eye
5. Relating to gold
6. ___uria; extravasation of urine
7. ___phobia; fear of light flashes
8. Innermost
9. To breast-feed
10. ___ pack; cold local application
11. U.S. hospital gp.
12. Dopamine transporter (acronym)
14. Without life
21. ___algia; chest pain
22. A bloodsucking aquatic annelid worm
25. ___itis; inflammation of the testes sac
26. A vivid mental picture
27. ___iasis; male hypersexuality
29. ___omosis; blood vessel coalescence
30. A network or plexus
32. ___tosis; prolapse of the large intestine
33. ___phobia; fear of the wind
34. Relating to the buttocks
35. ___taxis; slight hemorrhage
38. ___algia; toothache
39. Tumors (suffix)
40. Farther from the midline
45. A structure with comblike processes
46. A small pointed two-edged surgical knife
48. Any of various parasitic insects
49. The sole of the foot
50. The external opening of a space
51. Lip-shaped structures
52. Negatively charged ion
54. Prefix meaning 'eight'
55. The increase achieved by amplification of a signal
56. Computed tomography angiography (abbrev)
57. Automated external defibrillator (abbrev)
58. ___amnesia; false recollection

41

Across

1. ____ology; anatomy of the soft parts of the body
5. Instrument for recording (suffix)
10. Acute necrotizing ulcerative gingivitis (abbrev)
14. ____robic; without oxygen
15. ____rrhagia; ovarian hemorrhage
16. ____coid; scapular process
17. ____emia; presence of sodium in the blood
18. Relating to the ilium and vertebral column
20. To raise up
22. An infant aged 1 month or younger
23. ____ectomy; removal of the ileum
24. A line
25. Calcium salts in urine
32. ____ology; study of growth
33. Coagulated blood
34. Atrioventricular conduction (abbrev)
37. ____ogy; series of three
38. A youth
39. Abbreviation for N-formylglycinamide ribotide
40. Hepatitis A virus (abbrev)
41. A powerful oxidizing agent; O3
42. ____phobia; fear of religious or sacred objects
43. Digestive tract contractions
45. Abdominal distention
49. ____form; wing-shaped
50. ____tomy; incision of the lacrimal gland
53. An opening
57. A precursor
59. ____acusis; painful sensitivity to noise
60. To survey by traversing with a sensing device
61. Amyo____; muscle tone defect
62. Repose after exertion
63. Any weblike tissue
64. A condition of extreme distress
65. ____facient; causing movement

Down

1. Of sound mind
2. ____eptic; nervous system stimulant
3. Frequency of an event per unit of time
4. Referring to the neck
5. Thyroid gland enlargement
6. Behavior pattern individuals present to others
7. ____phobia; fear of bees
8. A unit of apparent loudness
9. A section of open-ended flexible tubing
10. Small saclike gland dilatations
11. Occurring on the 9th day
12. A salt of uric acid
13. ____ aponeurotica; epicranial aponeurosis
19. Being at opposite ends of a spectrum of values
21. ____ine; an amino acid
25. ____eter; fluid-removing body tube
26. Pre-migraine sensation
27. Roman 64
28. Thin serous discharge from a wound
29. ____ferous; conveying urine
30. Parameters for conduct or action
31. ____uria; urinary excretion of iodine
34. Grows older
35. ____cose; abnormally dilated
36. Acronym for contralateral routing of signal
38. Capillary zone electrophoresis (acronym)
39. Thread-like
41. Pertaining to sight
42. ____phagia; ingestion of an excessive quantity of salts
44. Dental calculus
45. Immature precursor cell (suffix)
46. Incise with a sharp object
47. Based on the number 8
48. ____virus; disease transmitted by rodents
51. ____morphosis; change of structure
52. ____toid; tooth-shaped
53. ____mania; compulsive shopping
54. ____phobia; fear of different mental conceptions
55. An enclosed fluid-filled sac
56. ____blast; a cell nucleolus
58. Electronystagmography (abbrev)

42

Across

1. Human antimouse antibody (abbrev)
5. Coagulation results
10. ___osis; drug-induced stupor
14. Enteropathogenic Escherichia coli (abbrev)
15. The pointed extremity of a structure
16. Eye, ear, nose and throat (abbrev)
17. 'Bridge' between medulla and midbrain
18. Referring to differences between ears
20. ___form; wing-shaped
21. Fibrous tissue connecting bones
22. Perceive flavour in the mouth
24. Nares
28. Ancient
31. Referring to a charged particle
32. Congenital displacement of any organ
36. Doctor of Physical Medicine (abbrev)
37. Lumbar puncture
41. Brinell hardness number (abbrev)
42. Connective tissue neoplasm
43. ___denitis; salivary gland inflammation
46. Referring to an apron
50. Half of a bilaterally symmetrical part
54. To tantalize
55. ___phobia; fear of neglect of duty
58. Mental telepathy (abbrev)
59. Science relating to human work
62. ___tia; denoting lack of force
63. ___osis; edema of bulbar conjunctiva
64. ___genic; causing cough
65. ___form; pea-shaped wrist bone
66. ___duct; seminal duct
67. Obstructive sleep apnea-hypopnea syndrome (abbrev)
68. Fetal alcohol spectrum disorders (abbrev)

Down

1. ___trophia; liver atrophy
2. Without polarity
3. ___ocyte; sickle cell
4. U.S. surgeons' society
5. Roman 902
6. Organ of respiration
7. Occurring every eighth day
8. ___phobia; fear of shaking
9. Any open skin lesions
10. ___phil; granular white blood cell
11. ___osis; production of gas in tissues
12. Carrier of genetic information (abbrev)
13. Cytotoxic T lymphocytes (abbrev)
19. Prefix meaning 'against'
21. To dissolve out by the action of a percolating liquid
23. ___itis; tendon sheath inflammation
25. ___genous; native to
26. Labia
27. A neck flexor (abbrev)
29. Inflammation of (suffix)
30. Source of cocaine
33. ___ anum; 'through the anus'
34. ___ordination; ataxia
35. Smallest unit of an element
37. ___algia; nose pain
38. ___omy; body structure study
39. ___genic; vomit-inducing
40. Of sound mind
41. Bovine serum albumin (abbrev)
44. Benign fatty tissue tumor
45. Acute motor axonal neuropathy (abbrev)
47. A coiled bandlike anatomic structure
48. Evaluate
49. Early cutaneous lesion of leprosy
51. ___genic; causing sexual arousal
52. An artery or nerve branch
53. Enzyme-linked immunosorbent assay (abbrev)
56. Interstitial cell-stimulating hormone (abbrev)
57. Upper attachment point for posterior sacroiliac ligament (abbrev)
59. Electrocardiogram (abbrev)
60. 17th letter of the Greek alphabet
61. ___eric; nonproprietary
62. Idiopathic pulmonary fibrosis (abbrev)

43

Across

1. Vessels in the body
5. A state of unarousable unconsciousness
9. ___ bifida; vertebral arch fusion failure
14. ___dotal; based on case histories
15. ___acusis; painful sensitivity to noise
16. ___cephalon; endbrain
17. The body of a nerve cell
18. Lowermost attaching structure
19. The external occipital protuberance
20. An adjustment that surpasses a set criterion
23. Negatively charged ions
24. U.S. surgeons' society
25. Clinical Laboratory Assistant (abbrev)
26. Fluorescence in situ hybridization (abbrev)
28. U.S. doctors gp.
31. Psychosis
34. The germinated and dried seed of barley
35. ___nestic; assisting the memory
36. Incision of the sclera and iris
39. ___rated; torn
40. Prefix meaning 'one trillionth'
41. ___gram; breast screening procedure
42. ___ment; constituent part
43. Roman 103
44. Abbrev. for complete blood count
45. Anodal opening contraction (abbrev)
46. Relating to the caudal transverse fissure
49. Within the adenoids
54. Acronym for disease modifying antirheumatic drugs
55. Roman 1155
56. ___thin; emulsifying phospholipid
57. Roman 903
58. ___olus; oxygen exchange pocket
59. Isopropylthiogalactoside (abbrev)
60. ___trum; initial breast fluid
61. Roman 59
62. Euthan___; mercy killing

Down

1. ___constriction; narrowing of blood vessels
2. Acronym for analysis of variance
3. Male ejaculatory fluid
4. Agent that destroys mites
5. An encircling structure
6. Smells or scents
7. ___rhexis; tearing of a muscle
8. ___brachium; forearm
9. A single suture
10. Male copulatory organ
11. ___psoas; hip flexor complex
12. Ne (chemical element)
13. ___ulus; ringlike structure
21. ___ptosis; prolapse of the vagina
22. ___ation; gonad removal
26. ___form; sickle-shaped
27. ___pexy; surgical fixation of ileum
28. ___aly; deviation from normal
29. ___algia; breast pain
30. ___esthesia; absence of muscle sensation
31. A tool for smoothing
32. Spoken
33. Small flat wingless parasitic insects
34. Roman 1102
35. Loss of the sense of touch
37. A figure-eight bandage
38. ___phobia; fear of rain
43. Of the heart
44. Evenly curved outward
45. ___megaly; enlargement of an atrium
46. Prefix referring to the basin-shaped hip structure
47. Lard
48. ___ferous; yielding milk
49. ___bilized; fixed
50. Protective cover on a dorsal distal phalanx
51. ___gam; cavity filler
52. Roman 655
53. ___ment; bone-connecting tissue
54. Roman 700

44

Across

1. Unable to hear
5. Suffix meaning 'killing'
10. Enteric cytopathogenic swine orphan (abbrev)
14. ___ology; study of feces
15. Expression of the relation of one quantity to another
16. Decays
17. Red blood cell destruction by isoantibodies
20. ___pyesis; suppuration in bone
21. Saliva
22. ___ectomy; removal of a vertebra
25. ___genetic; producing bile
26. ___virus; disease transmitted by rodents
30. ___ectomy; surgical removal of the uterus
33. Relating to feet
34. ___cus; hip flexor
35. ___dynia; shoulder pain
38. Production of insulin
42. Chief of Staff (abbrev)
43. ___ivore; flesh eating mammal
44. The soul or life
45. Loss of free-will ability
47. Olfactory organs
48. ___malacia; softening of the eye lens
51. Roman 152
53. Nervelike
56. Non-steroidal anti-inflammatory drug (abbrev)
60. Inflammation of tissues within the eyeball
64. Suffix meaning 'presence in urine'
65. ___denitis; salivary gland inflammation
66. Roman 602
67. Individual muscle unit
68. Squamous
69. Anterior border of tibia

Down

1. Roman 601
2. ___phobia; fear of dawn
3. ___taxis; slight hemorrhage
4. Worry
5. ___philic; preferring cold
6. ___rology; the science of medicine
7. Delayed-type hypersensitivity (abbrev)
8. Ventilates
9. Bend in a vessel forming a circular ring
10. ___algia; painful redness of the skin
11. ___genic; arising from a rib
12. ___born; born dead
13. ___ligamentous; made of bone and ligament
18. Remember
19. Small flat wingless parasitic insects
23. Nasal
24. Referring to the distal stomach aperture
26. ___otomy; incision into an apical structure
27. ___genic; originating in the kidney
28. Expanded disability status scale (abbrev)
29. ___pathia; seasickness
31. Something that causes an action
32. ___nia; coiled bandlike anatomic structure
35. Acid___; abnormally high acidity
36. Act out with gestures and body movement
37. Obstructive sleep apnea syndrome (abbrev)
39. Intensive care unit (abbrev)
40. Dwarfishness
41. ___phthalmos; recession of the eyeball
45. ___esthesia; loss of sensation of the limbs
46. Bronchiolitis obliterans with organizing pneumonia (abbrev)
48. ___atic; relating to gas or air
49. Unit of electrical inductance
50. ___genic; caused by sound
52. A graft into a cavity
54. Idiopathic hypertrophic subaortic stenosis (abbrev)
55. Dacarbazine (abbrev)
57. Immune system disease (abbrev)
58. Scratch trigger
59. Roman 503
61. Hepatitis-associated antigen (abbrev)
62. ___opath; traditional doctor
63. Breaking of moral law

45

Across

1. Wax
5. ___omia; inadequate body development
10. ___roma; artery wall mass
14. Toward the mouth
15. A minute fungus
16. ___cephalon; most recently evolved brain part
17. prefix meaning 'digest'
18. ___morphic; capable of assuming all shapes
19. ___emia; blood volume deficiency
20. Ultrasound image of the heart
23. ___ology; study of a cell's three-dimensional aspects
24. Salivary
25. B-type natriuretic peptide (abbrev)
27. Prefix meaning rose, red
31. Hepatitis-associated antigen (abbrev)
34. Inflammation of the peritoneal coat of the colon
39. ___esis; suppression of a discharge
41. Referring to the kidney
42. Sup. rectus femoris attachment pt.
43. Instrument for measuring muscular strength
46. Roman 102
47. ___phobia; fear of involuntarily shaking
48. Big clumsy person
50. Congenital absence of eye pupil
55. A thick fluid secretion
59. Having an inhibitory action on sweat secretion
62. ___phobia; fear of different mental conceptions
63. To give expression to feeling
64. Clinical Laboratory Improvement Amendments (abbrev)
65. ___itis; inflammation of a ligament
66. Saltpeter
67. U.S. OB/GYN gp.
68. ___gonist; something opposing the action of another
69. ___form; cartwheel-patterned
70. Narrow elevation of a bone

Down

1. Overcomes difficulties
2. Vertical in position
3. A seam of the halves of symmetrical parts
4. To take in or assimilate
5. ___cusis; hearing impairment
6. Time during which someone's life continues
7. ___culation; yawning and stretching
8. Small openings into hollow organs
9. Evacuated fecal matter
10. Congenital absence of the testes
11. Any weblike tissue
12. ___lich; abdominal thrust maneuver
13. Electronystagmography (abbrev)
21. Acronym for centromeric protein
22. A female youth
26. ___dynia; labor pains
28. Aural
29. Roman 503
30. ___form; resembling bone
31. ___ology; study of the structure of tissues
32. ___oid; star-shaped
33. Dull pain
35. Dream state (abbrev)
36. ___mia; decrease in red blood cells
37. ___gut; suture material
38. Prefix meaning 'oil'
40. A localized pool of blood
44. ___ceptor; receptor for pain
45. Artery or nerve branches
49. Forked
51. Unobstructs
52. To become less severe for a time
53. ___genic; causing sexual arousal
54. ___oid; resembling a star
56. ___ferol; vitamin D
57. The act of joining
58. A period in the course of a disease
59. ___algia; gland pain
60. A small mass of foreign cells
61. ___buccal; surrounding the cheek
62. Iminodiacetate (abbrev)

46

Across

1. A looplike structure
5. Coagulation results
10. ___phobia; fear of food or eating
14. ___itis; inflammation of the uterus
15. ___centesis; lumbar puncture
16. ___tia; denoting lack of force
17. ___sightedness; myopia
18. Muscle protein localized in the I band of myofibrils
19. Destitute of life
20. Between the transverse processes of the vertebrae
23. ___itis; inflammation of the lips
24. ___itis; blood vessel wall swelling
25. ___rhagia; hemorrhage from a breast
28. ___mania; over-talkativeness
30. ___phobia; fear of different mental conceptions
31. Small saclike gland dilatations
33. Epithelial membrane antigen (abbrev)
36. Elevation of body temperature by drug action
40. Unusual
41. Abnormal accumulation of interstitial fluid
42. Hairs
43. ___form; shaped like a wineskin
44. A significant life-changing event
46. ___algia; stomach ache
49. Pertaining to wild untamed animal
51. Regeneration of bone
57. ___itis; inflammation in the womb
58. Buttocks
59. ___plegia; paralysis of one limb
60. Bent (like a knee)
61. ___omosis; blood vessel coalescence
62. ___encephaly; abnormally small brain
63. The sum of all instincts for self-preservation
64. Periodically sheds an outer covering
65. Plant derived juice used on skin

Down

1. ___otic; fetus-surrounding fluid
2. ___cephalon; most recently evolved brain part
3. With no delay
4. That which raises
5. The most depressed central portion of an ulcer
6. ___mation; the secretion of tears
7. Relating to the number 8
8. Lean or slender
9. Breaks religious or moral laws
10. ___penia; iron deficiency
11. Deficient in active properties
12. To tantalize
13. A command or direction
21. 17th letter of the Greek alphabet
22. ___ectomy; colpectomy
25. ___chondria; energy producing organelles
26. Hyperactive child syndrome (abbrev)
27. Sperm
28. ___ment; bone-connecting tissue
29. A single
31. Angiotensin-converting enzyme inhibitors (abbrev)
32. Prefix meaning 'with'
33. Suffix meaning 'condition'
34. ___aria; heat rash
35. Lateral attachment of inguinal ligament (abbrev.)
37. ___dynia; pain in the uterus
38. Adverse drug reaction (abbrev)
39. The sheath covering a terminal nerve fibril
43. Womb
44. Bone ridges
45. Moved swiftly on foot
46. A strong
47. ___oid; resembling a star
48. ___cephaly; narrowness of the head
49. Causing death
50. To discharge waste
52. ___nestic; assisting the memory
53. Prefix meaning 'one billionth'
54. Dirt
55. ___ordination; ataxia
56. Tender

47

Across

1. ___lune; crescent shaped
5. Other licensed antifungal therapies
9. ___is; vocal apparatus of the larynx
14. ___cephaly; cranium defect with the brain exposed
15. Rate of movement
16. ___mation; the secretion of tears
17. ___aneus; heel bone
18. ___rhea; maintenance of water equilibrium
19. Muscle protein localized in the I band of myofibrils
20. Within a segment
23. ___ogen; female sex hormone
24. ___pose; fatty
25. Any enveloping structure
28. ___itis; joint 'sac' inflammation
30. Direct immunofluorescence (abbrev)
33. Rigid
34. ___algia; great artery pain
35. ___motor; moving the hair
36. Presence of calculi in the intestine
39. ___encephalon; forebrain
40. ___tis; inflammation of the large intestine
41. Structure resembling a bent bow
42. ___physis; a line of union
43. Shades or tints
44. Supporting framework of an organ
45. ___comenia; occurrence of menstrual ulcers
46. ___formis; external hip rotator
47. Resistant to cold
54. A benign neoplasm of muscular tissue
55. ___phobia; fear of forests
56. 9th letter in the Greek alphabet
57. A small cluster of cells
58. ___eurosis; sheet-like tendon
59. Away from the surface
60. ___cephaly; narrowness of the head
61. ___ilage; joint covering
62. End-stage renal disease (abbrev)

Down

1. ___bel; loudness measurement unit
2. ___thropic; originating outside the body
3. Denature
4. Grows in quantity
5. ___otic; behind the ear
6. Light beam device
7. U.S. OB/GYN gp.
8. A specified period of time
9. Substance secreting organs
10. ___ferous; yielding milk
11. ___valent; having a valence of eight
12. ___ogy; series of three
13. Sn (chemical element)
21. ___oid; resembling a star
22. Soil
25. Walking units
26. Unit of electrical inductance
27. ___ology; study of insects
28. Furuncles
29. ___caria; hives
30. ___pathy; intervertebral disc disease
31. The broad flaring portion of the hip bone
32. Hollow area of bone
34. Plant derived juice used on skin
35. The killing of one's parent
37. ___dynia; eye pain
38. ___liptics; treatment by inunction
43. ___colpos; retained menstruation
44. Producing no detectable signs or symptoms
45. Membrane across the virginal vagina
46. ___algia; distal stomach aperture pain
47. An enclosed fluid-filled sac
48. Behavior pattern individuals present to others
49. ___oid; lens-shaped
50. ___cusis; hearing impairment
51. Foot digits
52. A tubular passage
53. Continuous ambulatory peritoneal dialysis (abbrev)
54. ___anthropy; hatred of human beings

48

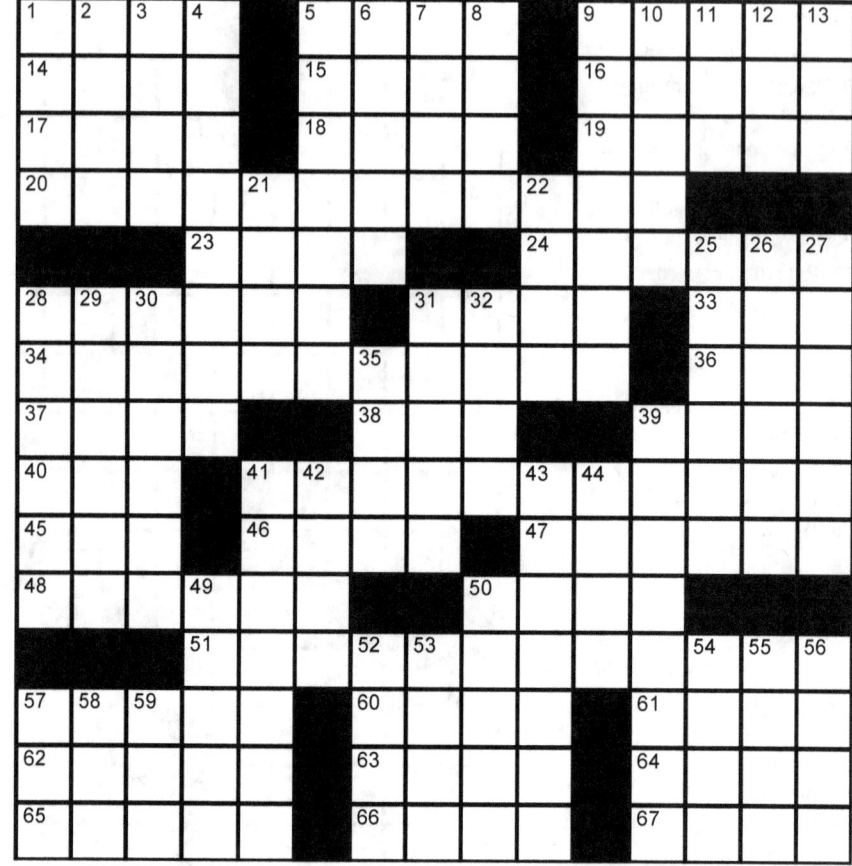

Across

1. Acetaminophen (abbrev)
5. Organ of respiration
9. Fast
14. Gangrenous stomatitis
15. Winglike structures
16. Excessively overweight
17. Adenosine deaminase acting on RNA (abbrev)
18. A thickening of skin on the toes
19. Movement of an organism to or from a stimulus
20. Relating to a single joint
23. Pb (chemical element)
24. Lack of muscle tone
28. SI units of magnetic flux density
31. Chicken embryo lethal orphan (virus)(abbrev)
33. A specific disease of sheep and goats
34. Agent used to hasten a chemical reaction
36. Direct immunofluorescence (abbrev)
37. ___itis; inflammation of a nipple
38. International Prognostic Index (abbrev)
39. To seal or fasten with wax or cement
40. Sn (chemical element)
41. Readily stained with osmic acid
45. ___ology; metaphysical study of the nature of being
46. ___emia; intestinal autointoxication
47. To induce recovery
48. Cytoplasmic body in the ovum that passes into the germ cell
50. Tender
51. A state of association
57. Crusts of superficial sores
60. Tunica
61. ___buccal; surrounding the cheek
62. Roman 952
63. Roman 1041
64. ___lary; referring to the armpit
65. Periodically sheds an outer covering
66. Enteroinvasive Escherichia coli (abbrev)
67. Ala ___; outside flaring wall of each nostril

Down

1. ___nestic; assisting the memory
2. ___dynia; foot pain
3. Acute motor axonal neuropathy (abbrev)
4. In the same plane but never meeting
5. Beta-galactosidase
6. Resembling a scar
7. ___osis; drug-induced stupor
8. Bent (like a knee)
9. A muscle that moves a bone around its own axis
10. ___gnosis; inability to sense weight
11. To fix or fasten
12. International sensitivity index (abbrev)
13. Diethylstilbestrol (abbrev)
21. Having verifiable existence
22. ___chezia; emotional discharge gained by swearing
25. A small palpable knot
26. Referring to iris inflammation
27. The feeling produced by a stimulus
28. To mark or colour the skin
29. ___cyte; burr cell
30. Odors
31. ___ulum; small head of a bone
32. ___tropic; directed against the cause
35. A cleft or crack
39. The duration of existence of an individual
41. The sense of smell
42. ___algia; leg pain
43. In front of the ear
44. ___iated; structure protruded through an opening
49. Eyeball socket
50. ___mesis; vomiting of saliva
52. Critical stage of a disease
53. ___phobia; fear of being poisoned
54. ___meric; containing six subunits
55. Rainbow-like eye part
56. Hairs
57. A neck flexor (abbrev)
58. Abbrev. for calculated mean organism
59. ___opath; traditional doctor

49

Across

1. Roman 1300
5. Acute inflammatory demyelinating polyradiculoneuropathy (abbrev)
9. Pertaining to sight
14. An organisms basic structural and functional unit
15. ___adenoma; benign sweat gland tumor
16. ___algia; pain in the sole of the foot
17. Plant derived juice used on skin
18. The compulsive eating of ice
20. Characterized by continuous tension
22. Deficient in active properties
23. Impregnated with a drug
26. Septic___; blood poisoning
30. Obstructive sleep apnea syndrome (abbrev)
31. Eyeing provocatively
33. ___able; deprive of capability
36. A group of three associated entities
39. ___form; lens-shaped
40. Adopting another's values as one's own
43. ___philia; voyeurism
44. Light beam device
45. ___algia; very severe pain
46. Process of eliminating a disease
48. ___oid; ring-shaped
50. Fetor ___; halitosis
51. A system of reasoning
56. A real or imaginary flat surface
58. To reduce to powder
60. Having but one layer
65. ___grity; soundness of structure
66. Rattling sounds in the lungs
67. ___itis; inflammation of a bone
68. Ne (chemical element)
69. Unobstructs
70. ___cephalon; most recently evolved brain part
71. Proximal upper limb parts

Down

1. Med. school applicant's test (abbrev)
2. The body cavity
3. A population of identical cells
4. Sterno_____mastoid; neck muscle
5. Viper or cobra
6. Isopropyl alcohol (abbrev)
7. Finger or toe
8. Face-down position
9. ___itis; eyebrow region dermatitis
10. Thrombocyte
11. Small outgrowth or polyp
12. ___encephaly; brain-exposing, occipital, cranial defect
13. Computed tomography angiography (abbrev)
19. ___dontics; pediatric dentistry
21. Smallest functional unit of heritability
24. ___ivore; flesh eating mammal
25. ___ism; absence of saliva
27. Fluid measure of about a drop of water
28. Metatarsus adductus
29. Growing older
32. Fixedly and angrily staring
33. ___pathy; intervertebral disc disease
34. ___vation; a bending inward
35. ___form; cartwheel-patterned
37. Wing-like process
38. Rounded flat plates
41. ___itis; inflammation of the capsule of the spleen
42. Absence of all quantity or magnitude
47. Metric unit of weight
49. A ridgelike structure
52. Negatively charged ion
53. Rigid
54. An internal layer of protective material
55. ___ology; study of insects
57. ___itude; a sense of weariness
59. A toothlike structure
60. ___dynia; pain on urination
61. Snooze
62. ___ectomy; removal of the ileum
63. Had food
64. kidney

50

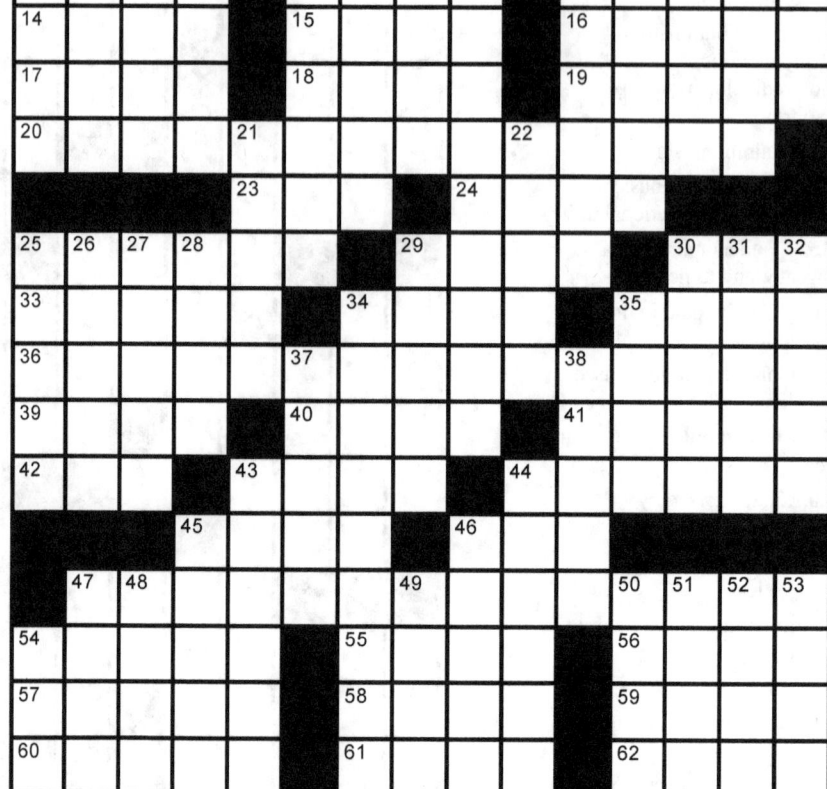

Across

1. A pointed end
5. ___constriction; narrowing of blood vessels
9. A salt of uric acid
14. ___itis; inflammation of the female gonad
15. Enzyme-multiplied immunoassay technique (abbrev)
16. Bubbling sounds in the lungs
17. ___derma; atrophic skin of the aged
18. ___genic; originating in the kidney
19. Surface borders
20. Sleepwalking
23. Mini stroke (abbrev)
24. ___ology; study of dreams
25. Thin specimens for examination
29. N-formylglycinamide ribotide (abbrev)
30. Adult male
33. Spheroid bacteria
34. Fetor ___; halitosis
35. ___ cava; main vein
36. Appliance used to manage prosthetic problems related to tooth alignment
39. Minute opening of the skin
40. ___algia; homesickness
41. Anal injection of fluid
42. ___matomania; abnormal impulse to dwell on certain words
43. Gamete intrafallopian transfer (abbrev)
44. Pertaining to the backbone
45. A fold, ridge, or crease
46. ___enuate; to diminish
47. Agent that causes vomiting and purging
54. ___osis; failure of ossification
55. ___grity; soundness of structure
56. ___genesis; the formation of gas
57. A drop
58. ___esia; no movement
59. ___ogy; series of three
60. Irregularly notched
61. ___pene; red pigment of a tomato
62. Prefix meaning 'delight in cruelty'

Down

1. ___ition; the process of knowing
2. ___scleritis; scleritis due to uveitis
3. ___ology; anatomy of the soft parts of the body
4. ___ract; to extend forward
5. A wormlike structure
6. Single-celled organism (variable)
7. ___atrial node; pacemaker
8. Specialist of conditions and diseases of the ear
9. Tube that carries urine from the kidney to the bladder
10. Lateral forearm bones
11. ___genic; producing pain
12. Puberty person
13. Feminine suffix
21. ___megaly; enlargement of an atrium
22. ___omosis; blood vessel coalescence
25. ___philia; voyeurism
26. A stupid person
27. ___geny; congenital absence of a body part
28. Dull pain
29. Deposit resembling that of frozen vapor
30. ___cephalon; midbrain
31. The soul or life
32. Pertaining to the nose
34. Relating to the mouth and face
35. ___puncture; surgical puncture of a vein
37. ___phobia; fear of choking or smothering
38. Prefix meaning 'seven'
43. Drops
44. ___metry; measurement of muscular strength
45. Relaxes
46. Epitympanic recess
47. ___esis; involuntary discharge of urine
48. ___facient; causing movement
49. ___losis; fusion of a joint
50. Disease-spreading rodents
51. Prefix signifying one trillion
52. ___ectomy; excision of part of the iris
53. Prefix meaning 'large intestine'
54. Life time

Medi-Cross III

ANSWERS

1

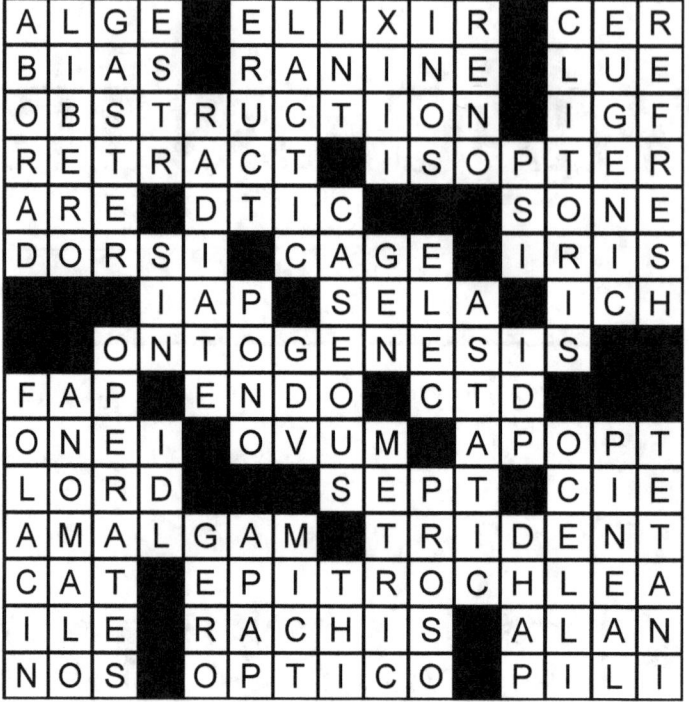

2

3

H	E	A	T	S		S	C	E	L		L	A	M	P
O	C	T	E	T		T	O	X	I		I	R	I	S
C	H	O	L	E	C	Y	S	T	E	C	T	O	M	Y
M	O	M	E	N	T			E	N	D	E	M	I	C
			T	A	L	A	R			A	R	A	C	H
T	A	L	I		A	M	N	I						
A	N	A	P	H	A	S	E		D	C	C	C	X	C
P	A	N	T	A	N	E	N	C	E	P	H	A	L	Y
S	T	I	G	M	A		T	R	O	P	O	N	I	N
			L	E	I	O			L	E	V	O		
A	V	I	A	N		N	A	S	A	L				
N	E	C	R	O	S	E		N	E	V	O	I	D	
I	N	T	E	R	T	R	A	N	S	V	E	R	S	E
S	T	U	N		A	G	U	E		I	N	I	O	N
O	S	S	A		T	Y	R	O		T	E	S	T	S

4

O	P	S	I		D	E	A	F		L	A	B	R	A
L	A	W	S		M	X	L	I		I	N	I	A	C
I	L	E	O	C	E	C	A	L		P	O	L	Y	P
V	I	L	L	I		R	E	T	I		M	A	S	S
E	N	L	A	R	G	E		H	E	M	A	T		
			T	R	E	M	O		P	I	L	E	U	S
L	A	S	E		N	E	S	T		T	O	R	T	I
E	M	T		P	E	N	T	O	S	E		A	R	T
S	P	A	C	E		T	E	L	A		I	L	I	O
B	U	B	O	E	S		M	E	D	I	A			
			I	N	L	E	T		R	O	S	T	R	A	L
L	A	L	I		P	A	B	A		O	R	E	X	I
U	R	I	C	O		P	A	N	O	T	I	T	I	S
N	O	T	A	N		H	D	C	V		C	R	O	S
A	M	Y	L	O		O	L	E	O		S	O	N	O

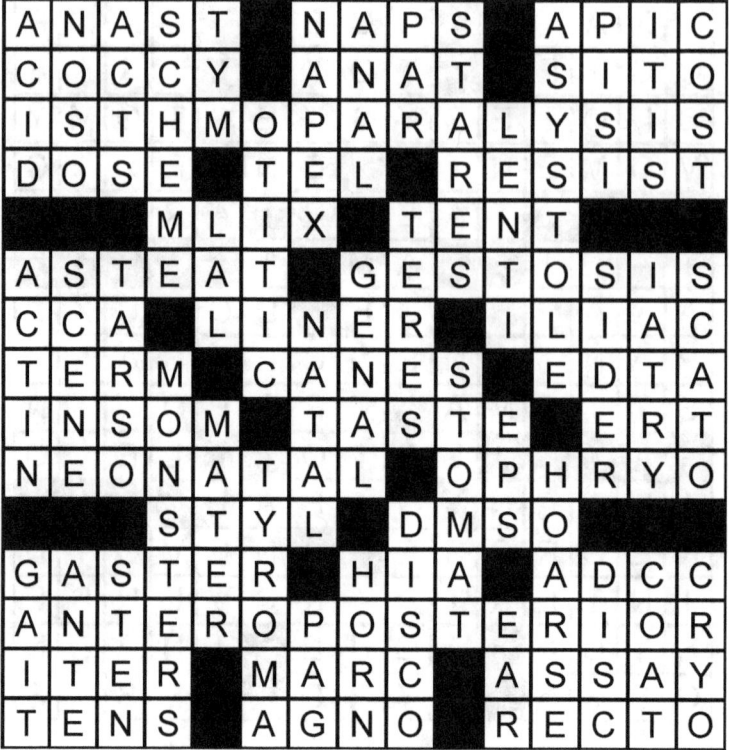

7

O	A	T	H		L	A	M	E		O	S	T	I	A
A	U	R	I		I	D	E	A		S	T	I	L	L
F	R	O	S	T	B	I	T	E		T	E	N	I	A
S	A	C		H	E	P	A		M	O	R	T	A	R
			H	I	E	R	O		D	O	S	E		
P	H	A	L	L	O		P	E	R	I	O	D	I	C
S	A	N	I	O		R	A	L	E	S		I	N	H
O	N	T	O		M	E	L	T	S		O	S	S	I
A	D	E		G	E	M	M	A		E	C	T	A	L
S	I	R	I	A	S	I	S		E	X	T	E	N	D
			O	L	A	T		A	V	I	A	N		
C	A	U	D	A	D		A	N	E	S		T	H	I
A	T	T	I	C		A	C	A	N	T	H	I	O	N
C	H	E	S	T		N	E	S	T		C	O	R	N
H	E	R	M	A		T	I	T	S		I	N	I	O

8

C	R	I	B		C	O	C	A		C	L	A	S	P
M	E	N	O		A	N	A	P		H	I	R	C	I
I	N	T	R	A	P	E	R	I	T	O	N	E	A	L
V	I	R	A	L		I	N	C	O		C	A	R	O
			G	V	H	R		A	N	A	T			
F	A	C	E		F	O	L	L	I	C	U	L	A	R
L	D	L		L	V	I	X		C	A	R	I	N	A
A	R	E	N	A		D	X	L		R	E	N	I	N
R	E	F	E	C	T		V	I	V	O		E	O	G
E	N	T	O	R	E	T	I	N	A		C	A	N	E
			P	I	L	E		I	L	E	O			
S	C	E	L		A	N	A	M		T	R	A	P	S
N	O	T	A	N	E	N	C	E	P	H	A	L	I	A
A	N	I	S	O		I	N	N	O		C	A	R	D
P	S	O	M	O		S	E	T	S		O	N	I	O

9

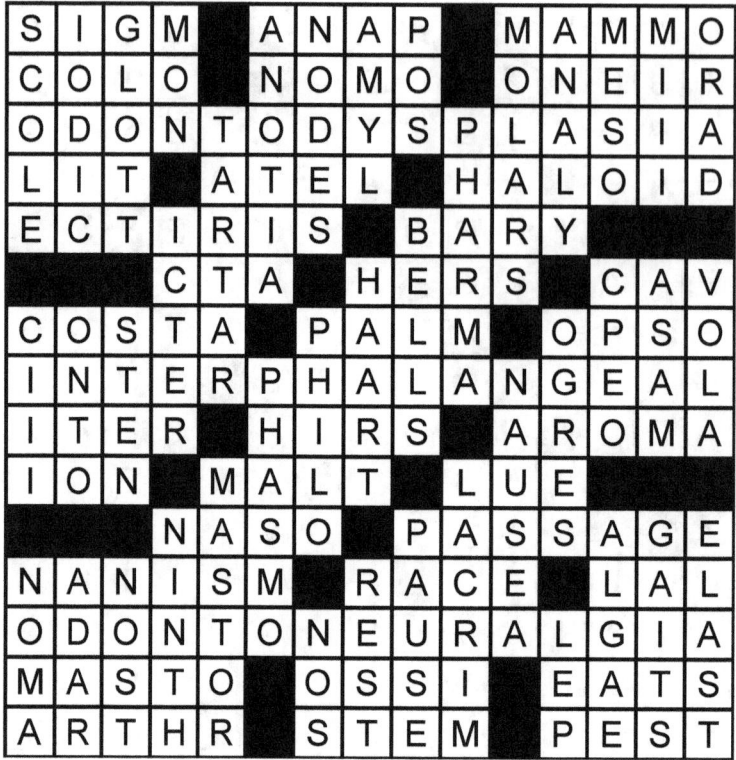

10

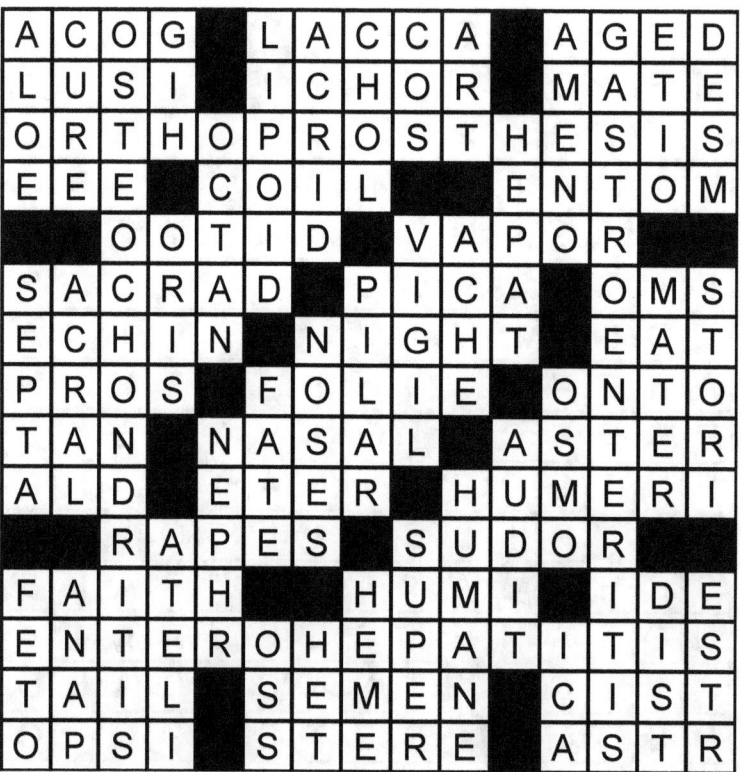

11

E	L	B	O	W		I	T	C	H		P	H	O	T
L	O	U	P	E		S	E	M	I		R	E	T	I
E	X	C	I	T	O	M	E	T	A	B	O	L	I	C
C	O	C	A		R	U	N		T	U	N	I	C	S
			T	A	G	S		V	A	S	A			
A	M	O	E	B	A		C	A	L		T	A	L	I
S	A	C		A	S	C	U	S		B	O	N	E	S
I	N	T	E	R	M	E	T	A	T	A	R	S	A	L
A	G	A	M	O		C	A	L	O	R		A	R	E
L	E	N	I		C	A	N		P	O	T	E	N	T
		C	O	L	L		D	O	T	E				
G	L	O	T	T	O		D	I	G		C	O	A	T
R	E	G	I	O	N	A	L	A	N	A	T	O	M	Y
A	C	R	O		I	T	I	S		L	A	Z	A	R
D	I	E	N		C	L	I	T		G	L	E	N	O

12

A	C	I	D		T	A	L	A	R		A	R	C	H
D	M	S	O		A	N	I	M	A		C	O	L	E
P	H	O	T	A	U	G	I	A	P	H	O	B	I	A
	C	R	E	S	T		N	E	U	R	O	I	D	
			S	O	M	A		M	I	T	I	S		
T	R	I	B	E		A	M	E	L	I	A			
H	E	A	T	S		N	A	S	I		A	N	A	
I	N	T	U	S	S	U	S	C	E	P	T	I	O	N
N	O	R		P	A	T	H		H	E	L	C	O	
		A	L	A	L	I	A		R	A	D	I	X	
U	V	U	L	A		A	R	T	I					
R	E	L	A	X	E	S		A	N	A	S	T		
I	N	T	R	A	C	E	R	E	B	E	L	L	A	R
N	O	R	M		S	T	A	T	O		K	I	L	O
O	M	A	S		O	S	M	I	O		A	T	O	M

13

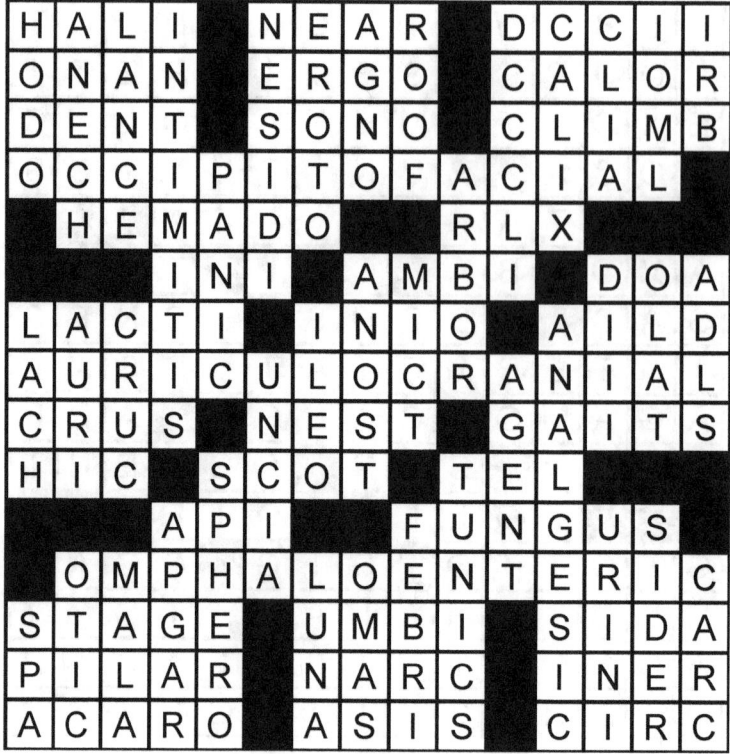

14

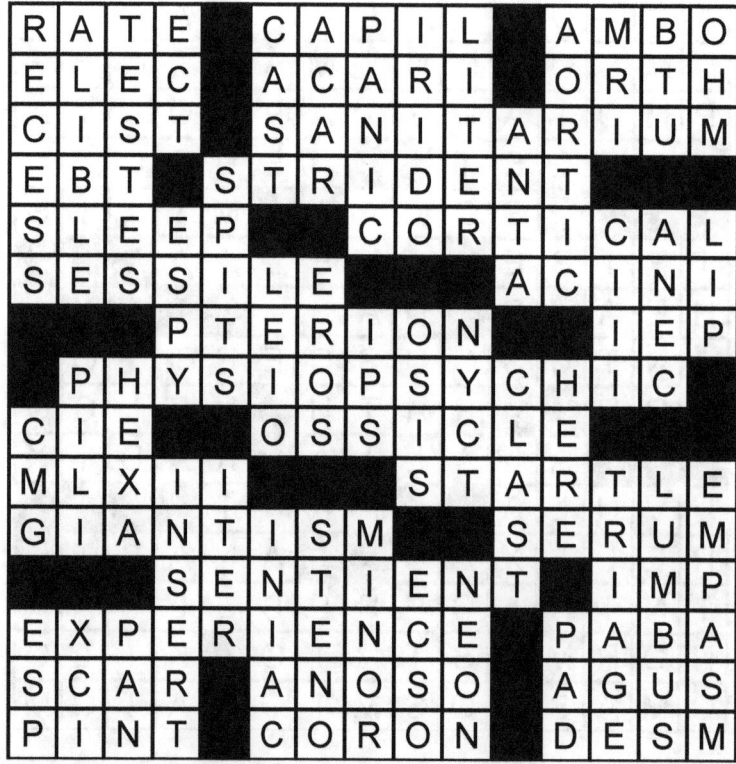

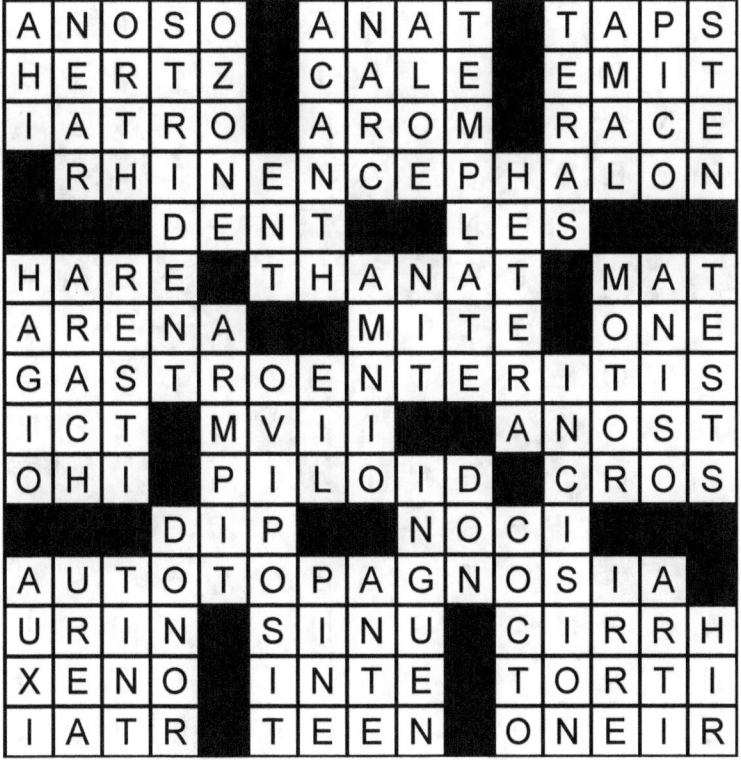

17

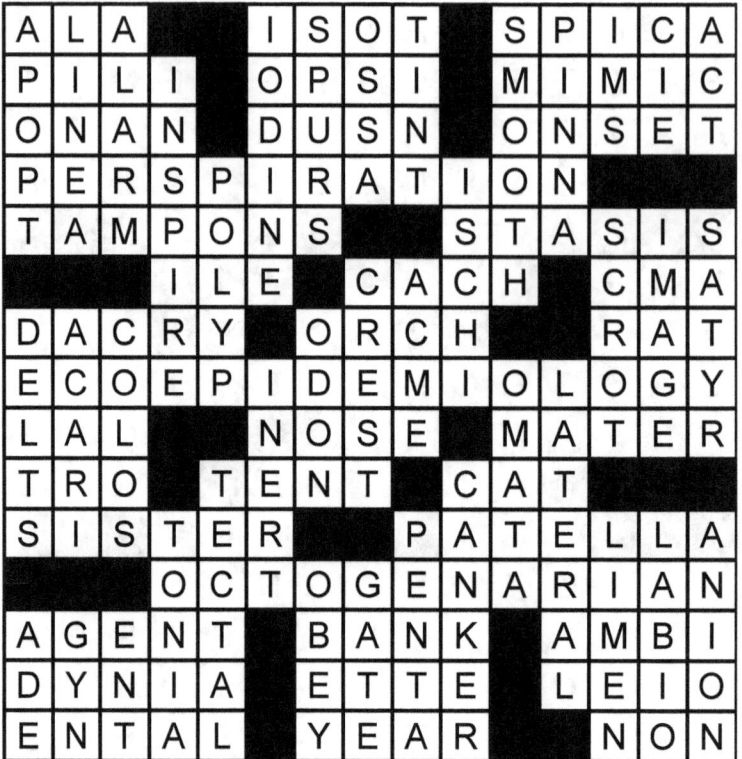

18

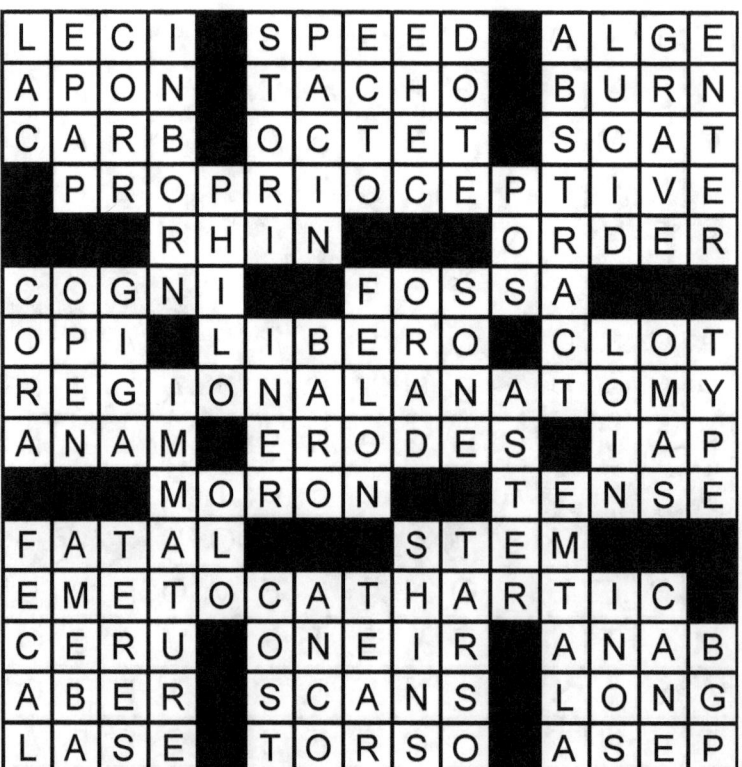

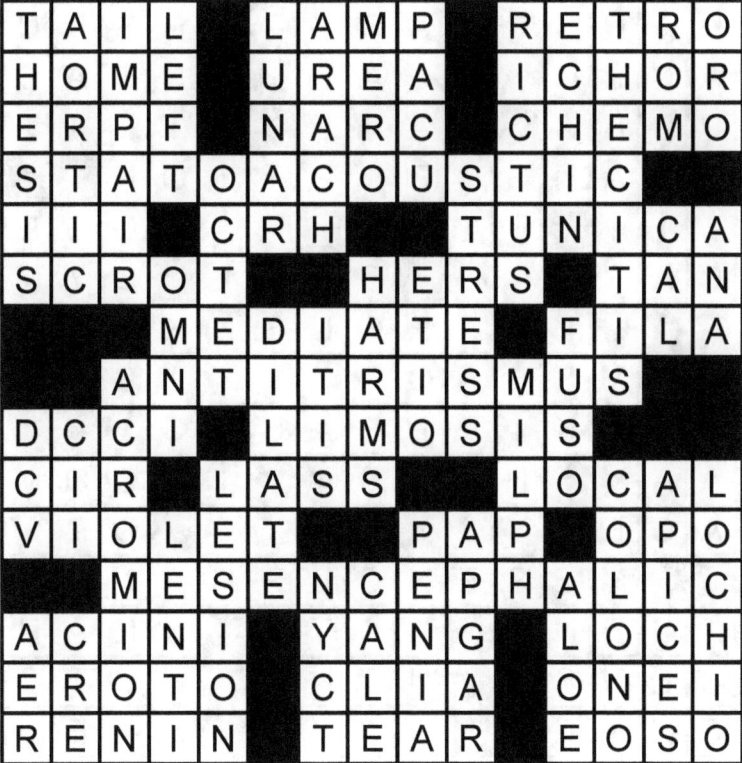

21

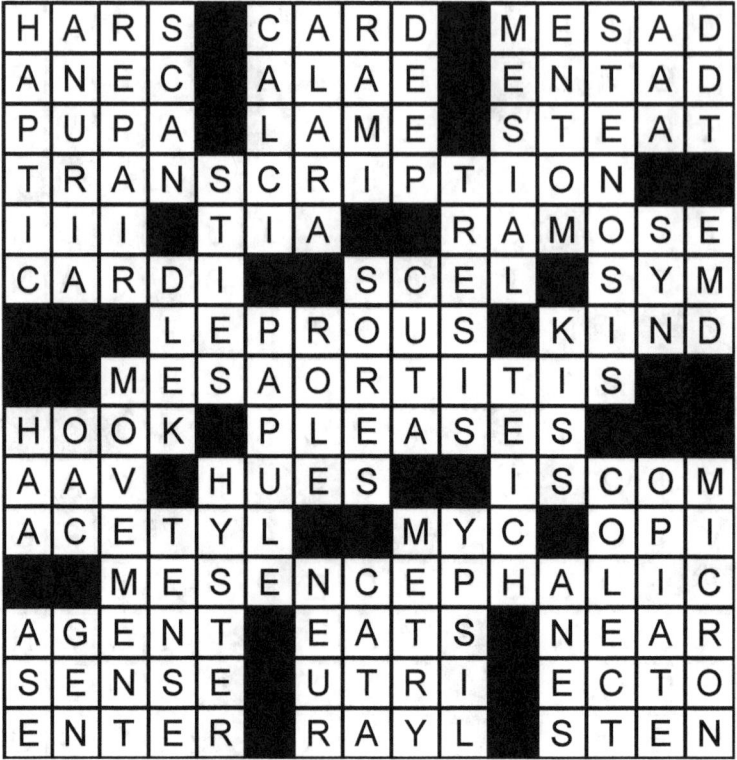

22

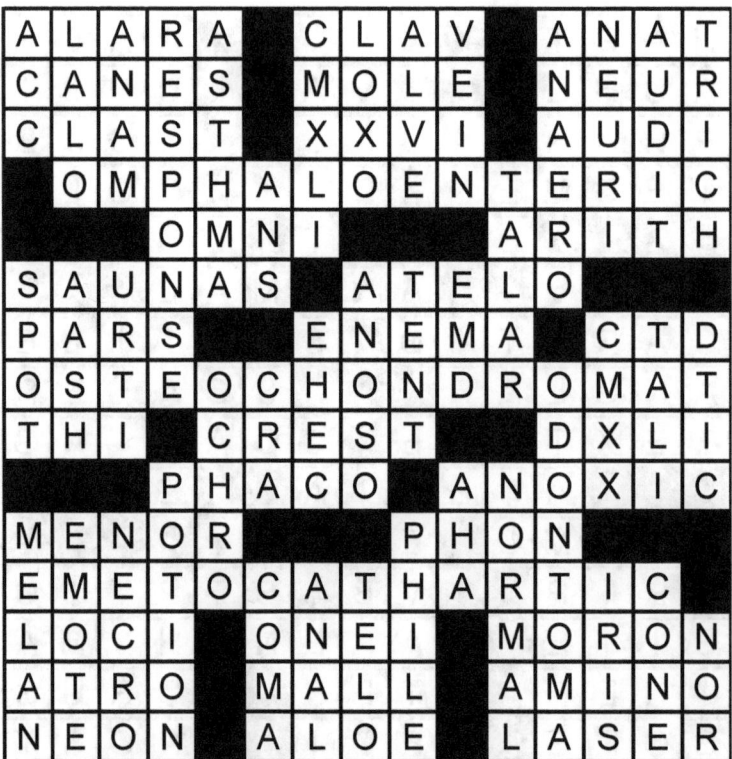

23

A	T	R	O		C	O	A	P	T		D	T	P	A
U	R	I	C		A	G	G	E	R		T	H	E	C
T	A	C	T		U	R	I	N	E		P	A	R	O
I	N	T	E	R	D	E	N	T	A	L		N	A	U
S	C	A	T	O			G	A	T	E		A	N	S
M	E	L		B	A	L			S	P	U	T	U	M
				M	O	B	I	L	E		N	O	M	A
			N	A	T	R	I	U	R	E	S	I	S	
	C	R	U	C		I	M	P	A	C	T			
	R	E	T	R	A	D		F	E	L		A	D	H
	I	L	A		M	E	T	A		E	C	T	R	O
	C	A	T		P	R	O	C	T	O	R	R	H	E	A
	O	P	I	A		M	O	U	R	N		Y	E	A	R
	I	S	O	R		A	T	T	I	C		A	R	M	S
	D	E	N	T		T	H	E	L	O		N	O	S	E

24

R	A	G	E		M	A	S	S		M	U	R	A	L
A	N	E	S		U	N	C	I		O	V	A	R	I
C	A	R	T		S	E	A	T		L	U	M	E	N
H	E	M	I	E	C	T	R	O	M	E	L	I	A	
			M	E	L	O			C	C	A			
S	C	I	A	G	E		P	A	C	U		S	T	Y
T	A	C	T			C	A	P	I	L		T	A	P
A	R	T	E	R	I	O	L	O	V	E	N	O	U	S
I	B	U		E	D	G	E	S		A	R	T	I	
N	O	S		G	E	N	O		V	A	R	I	O	L
			B	N	A		M	I	S	C				
	P	A	R	A	L	I	P	O	P	H	O	B	I	A
O	R	G	A	N		C	A	N	E		S	A	R	C
S	O	N	I	C		D	I	A	R		I	S	O	T
A	G	O	N	Y		A	R	D	S		S	I	N	S

25

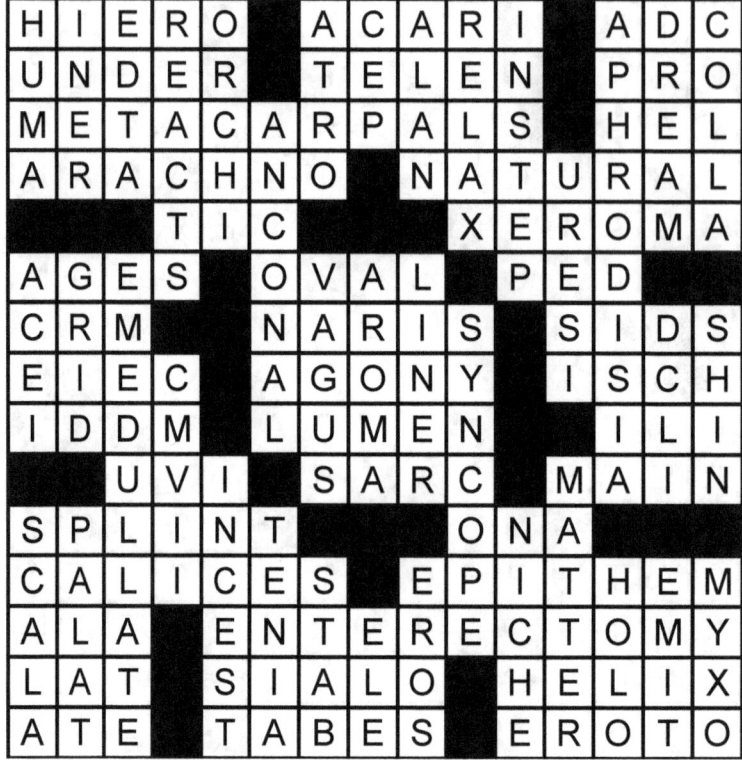

26

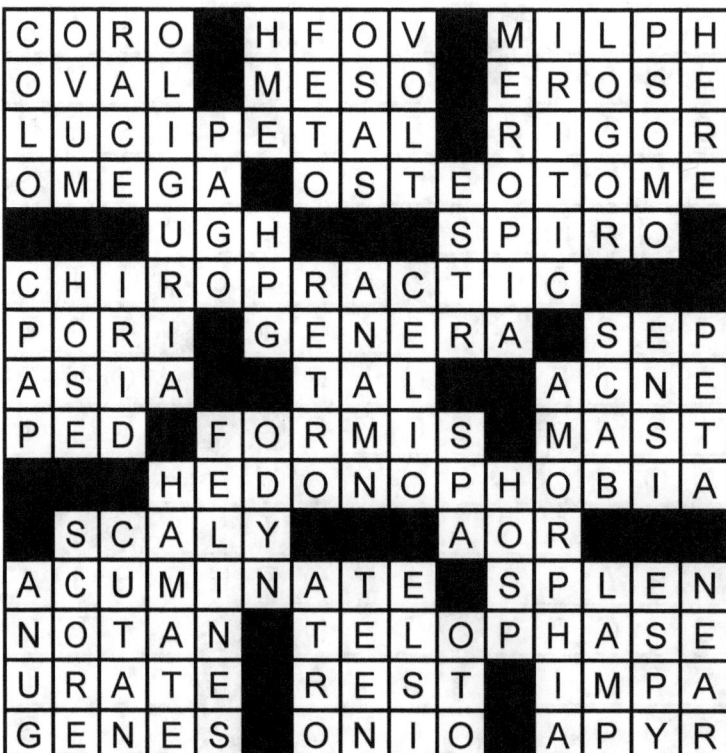

27

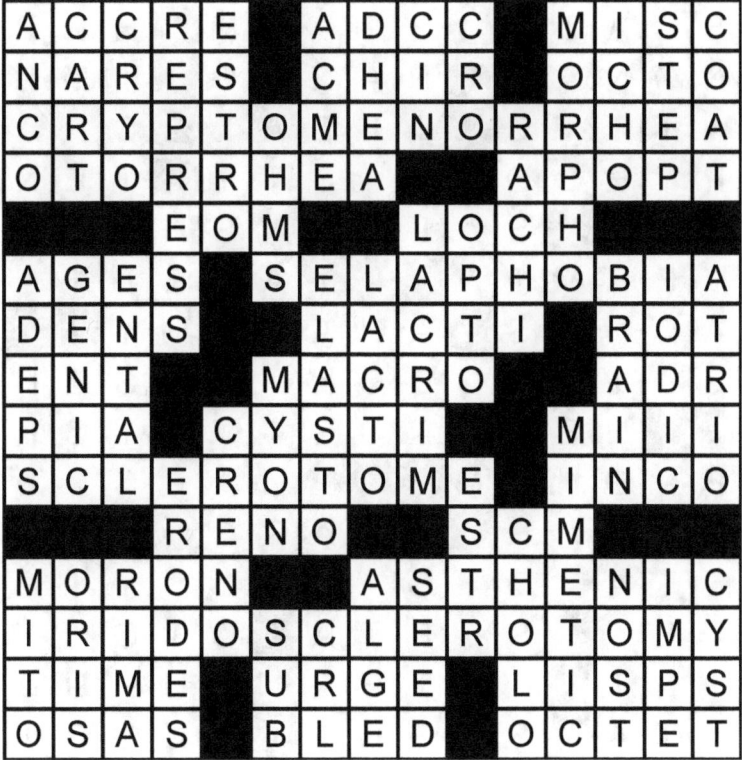

28

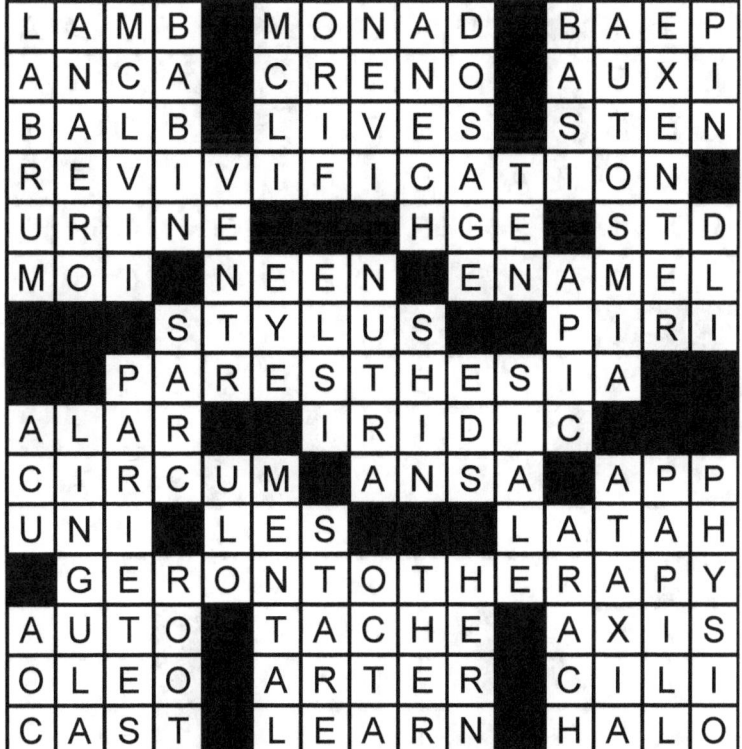

29

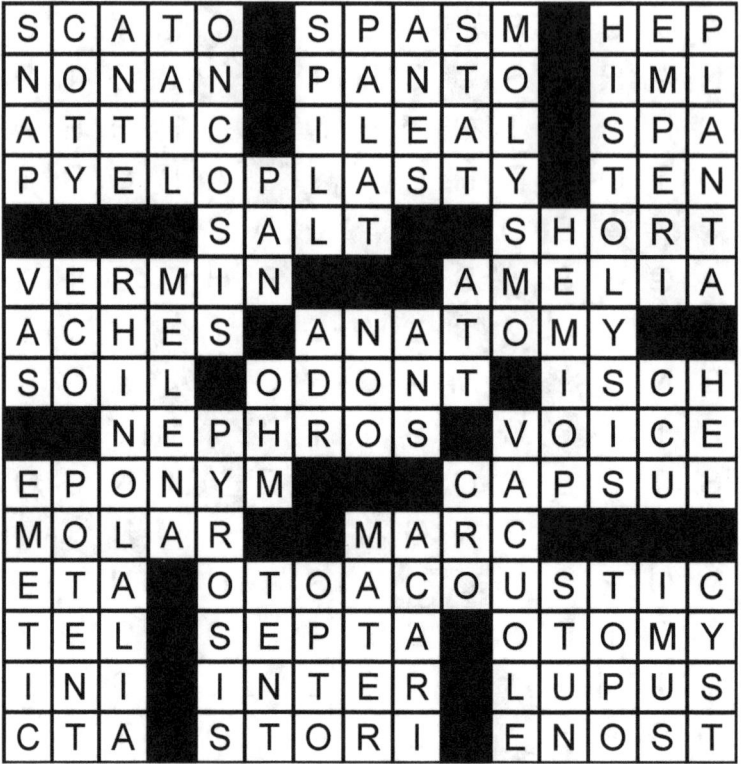

30

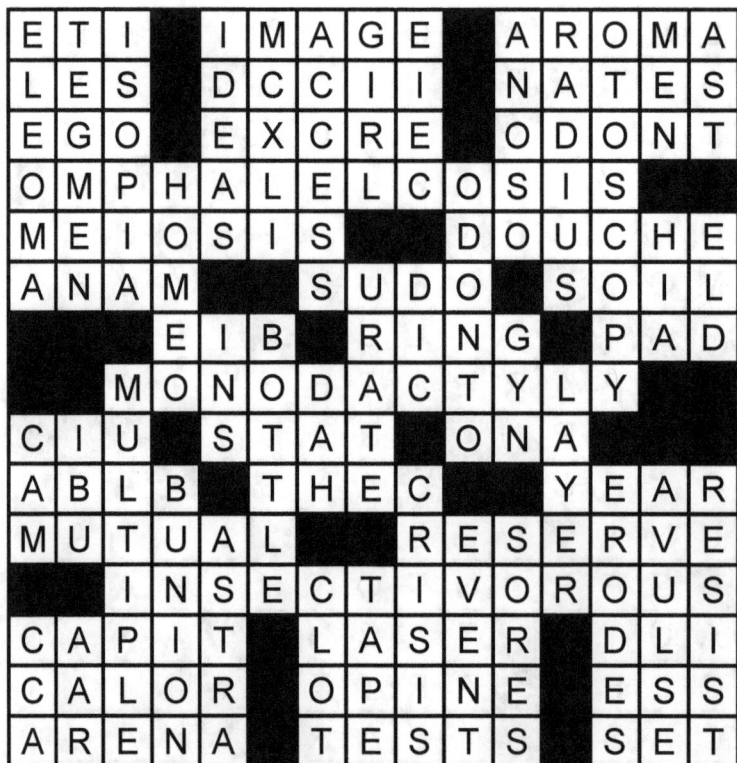

31

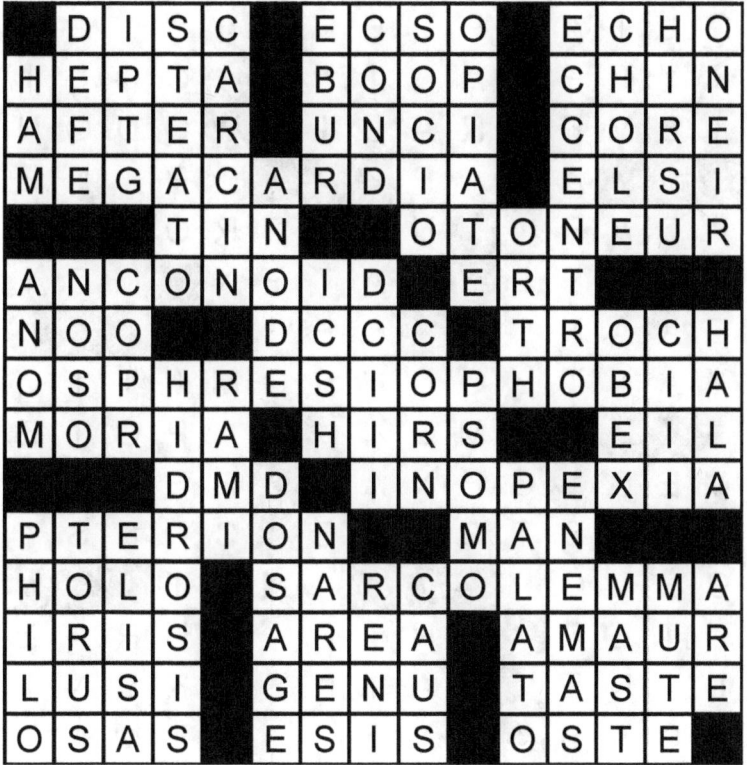

32

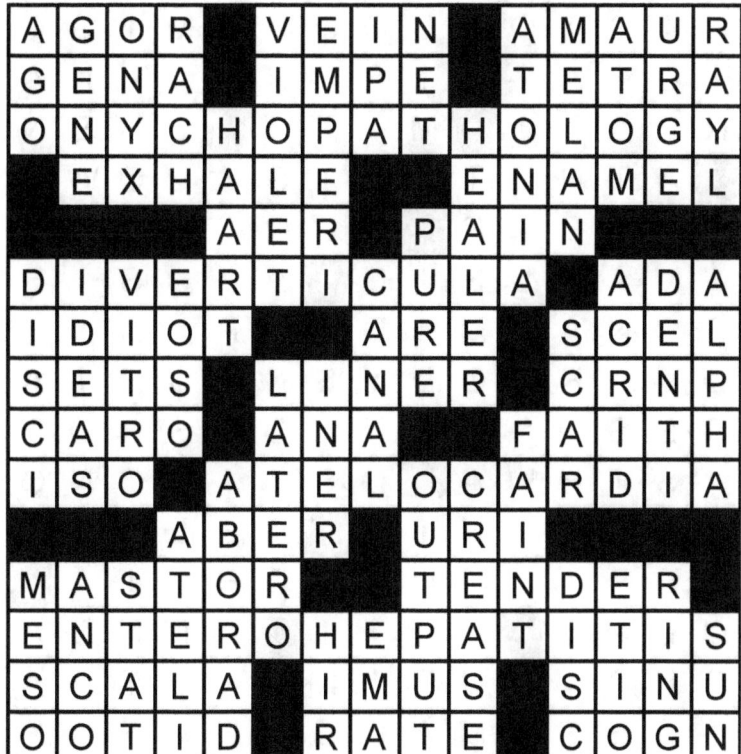

33

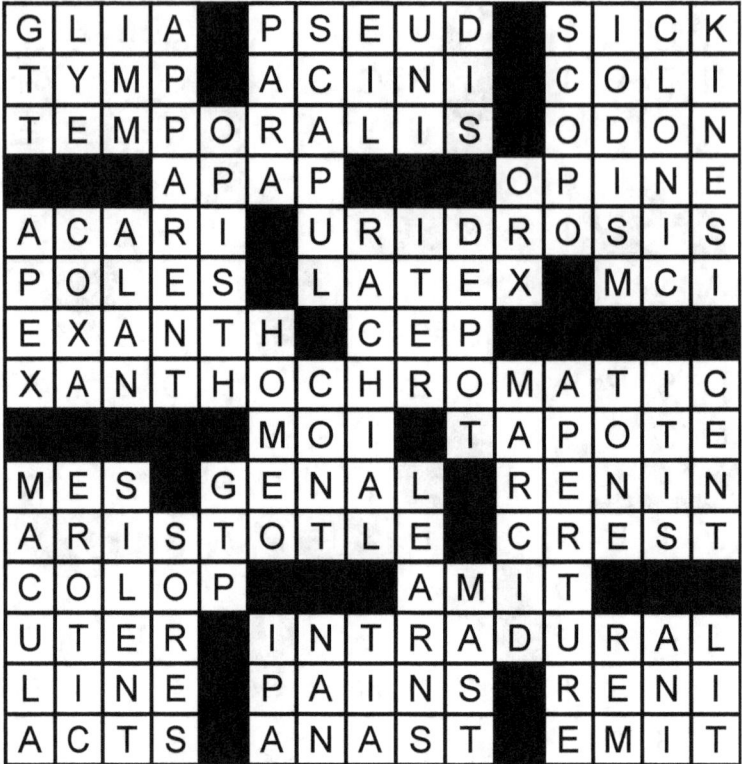

34

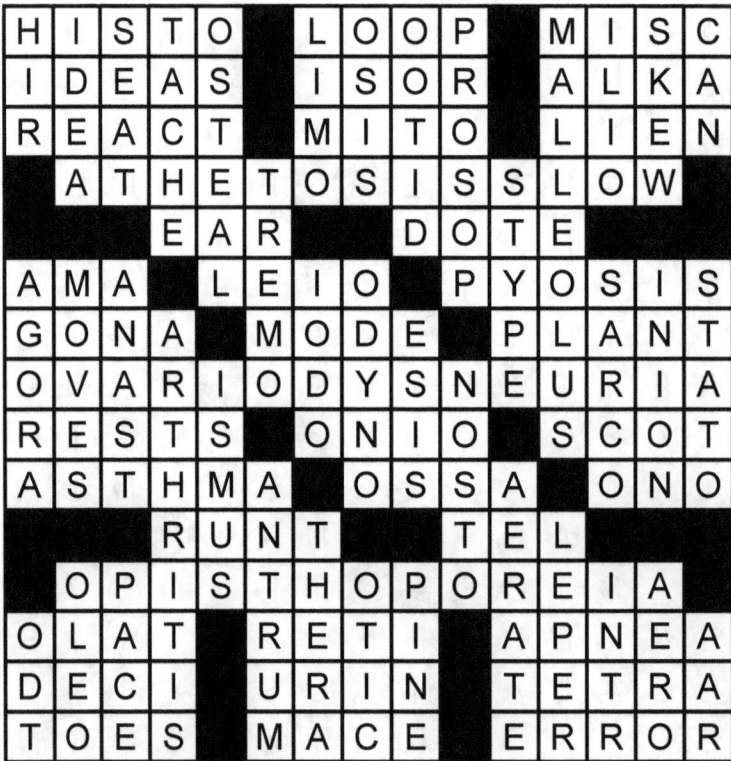

35

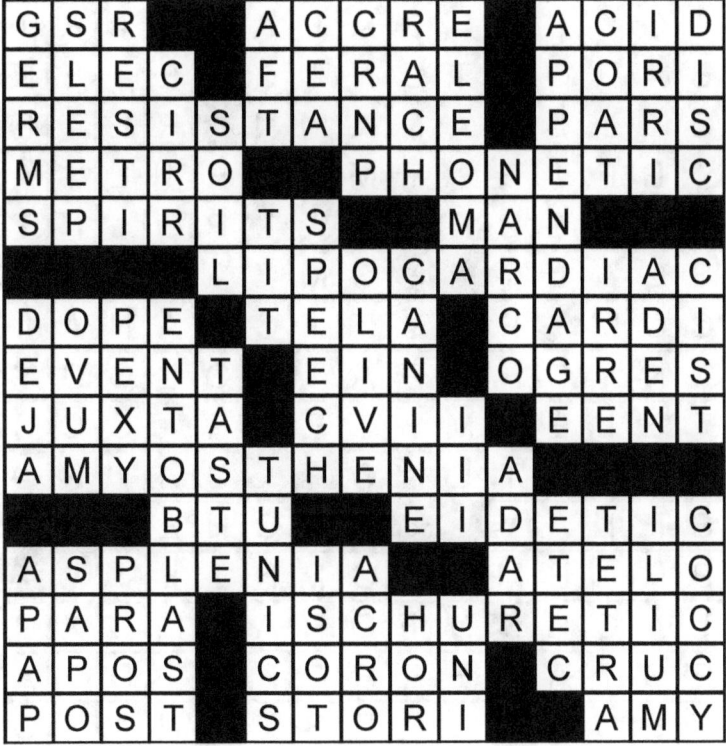

36

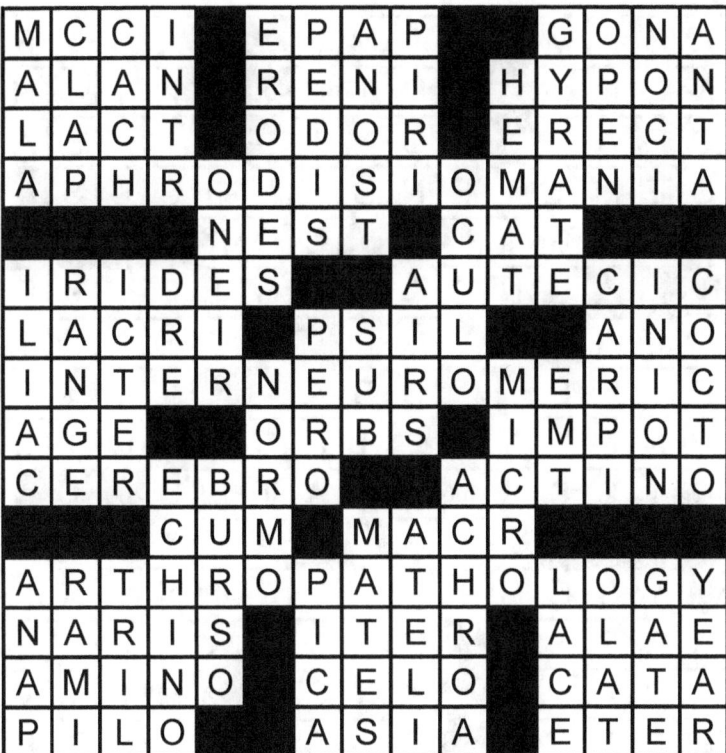

37

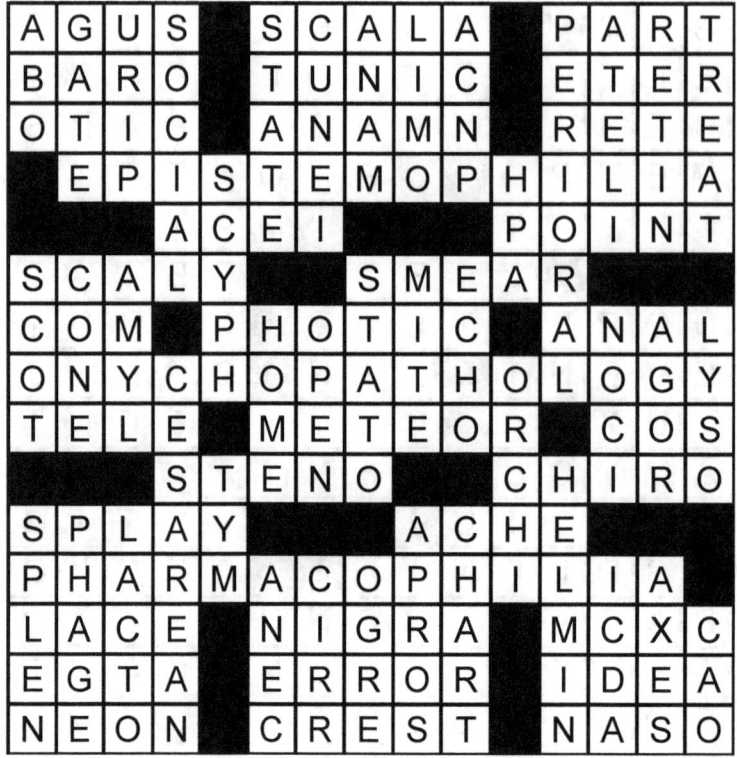

38

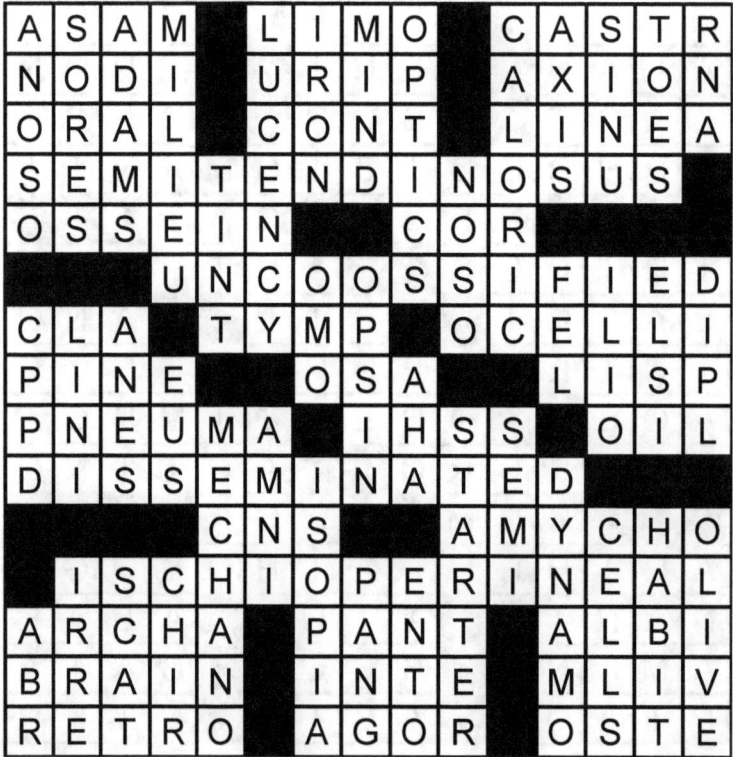

39

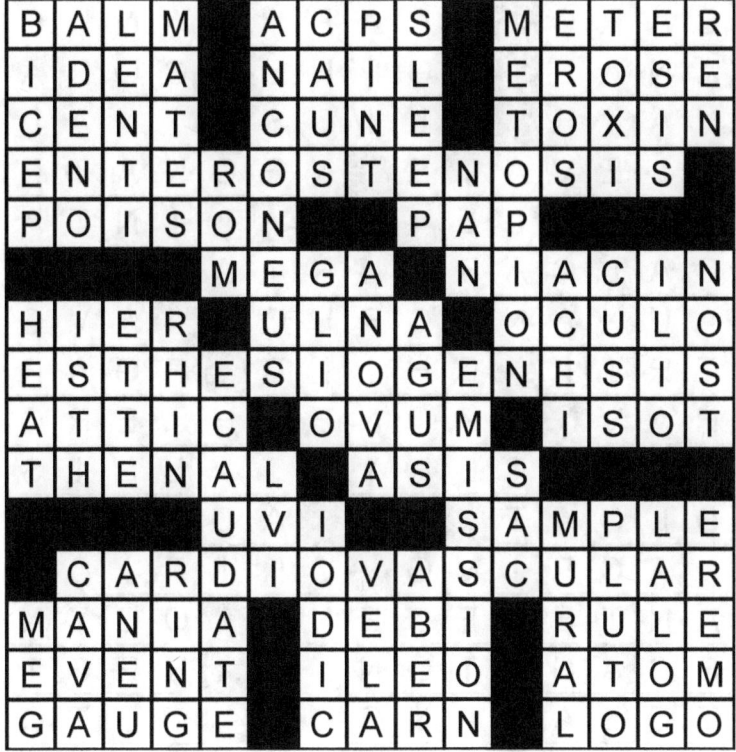

40

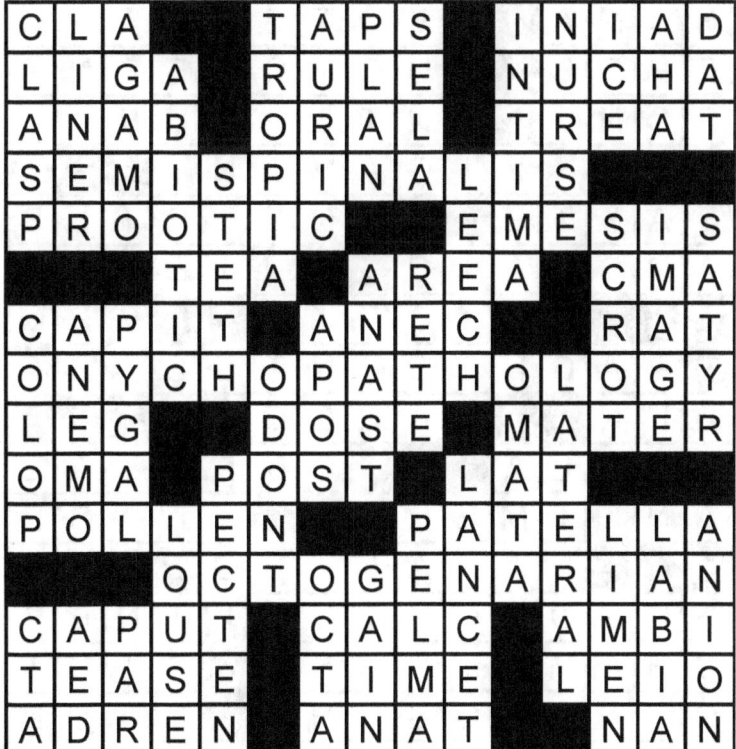

41

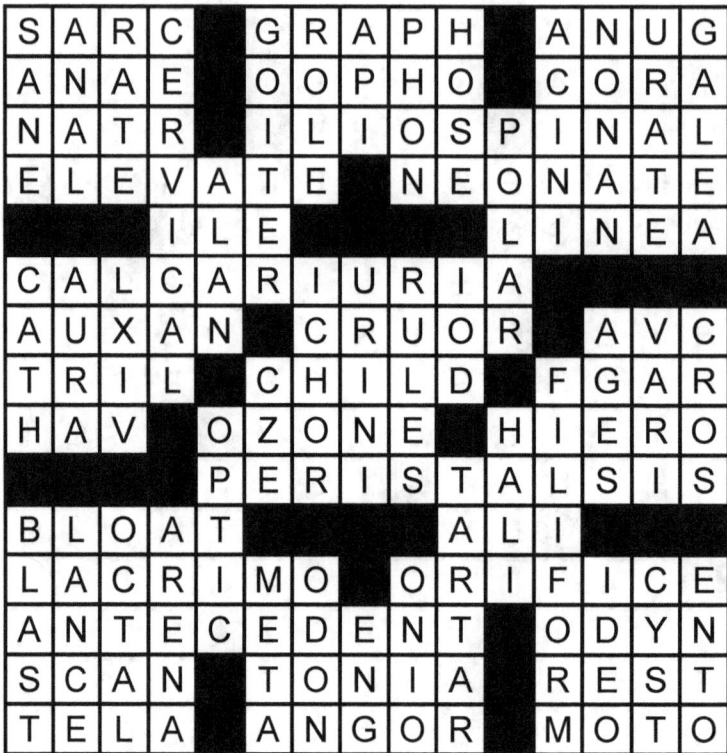

42

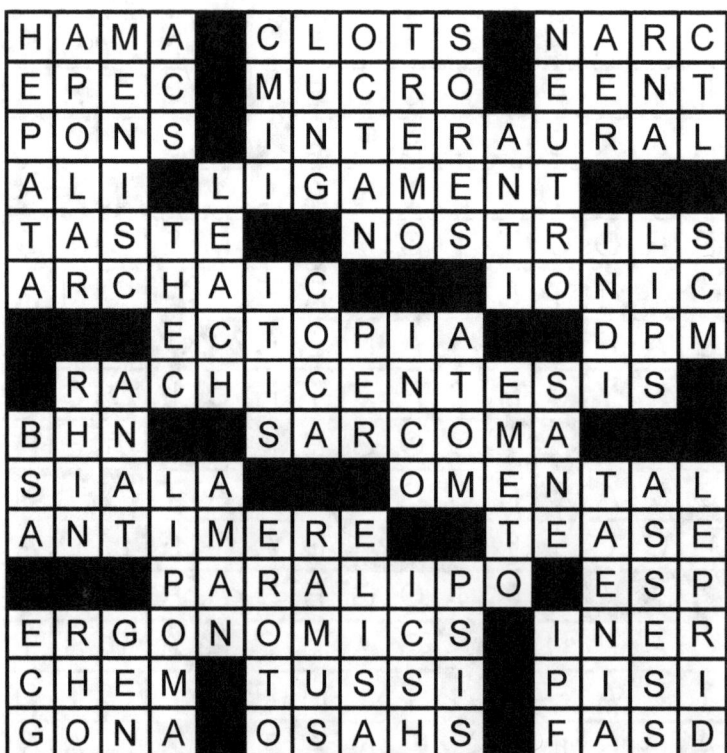

43

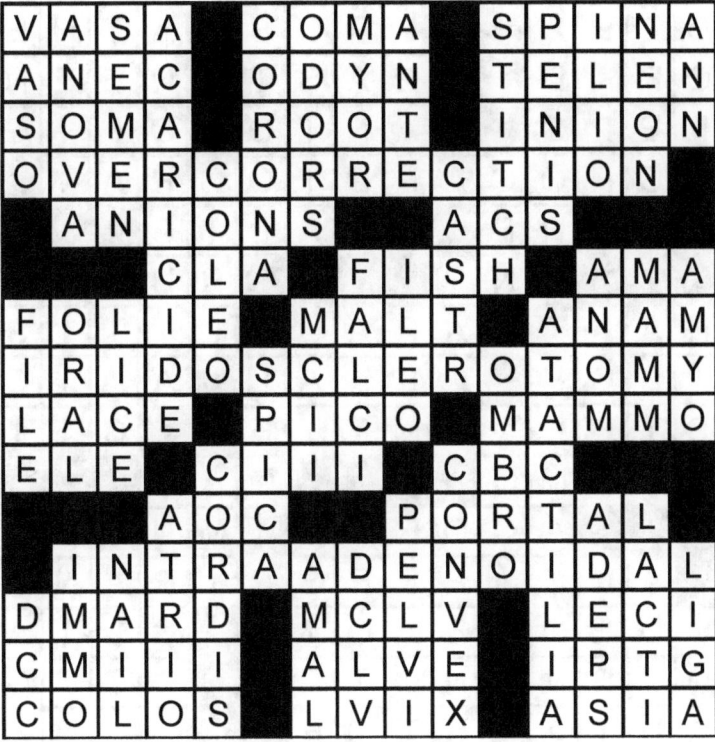

44

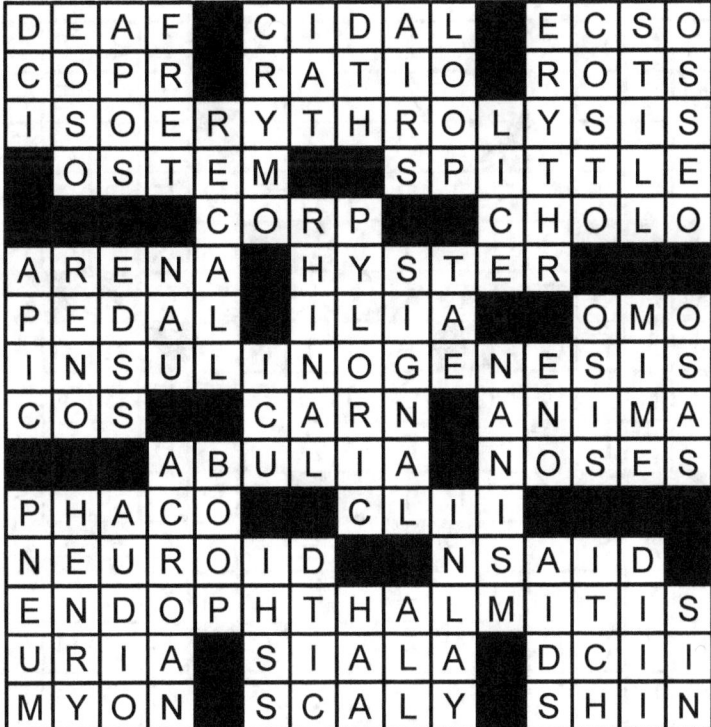

45

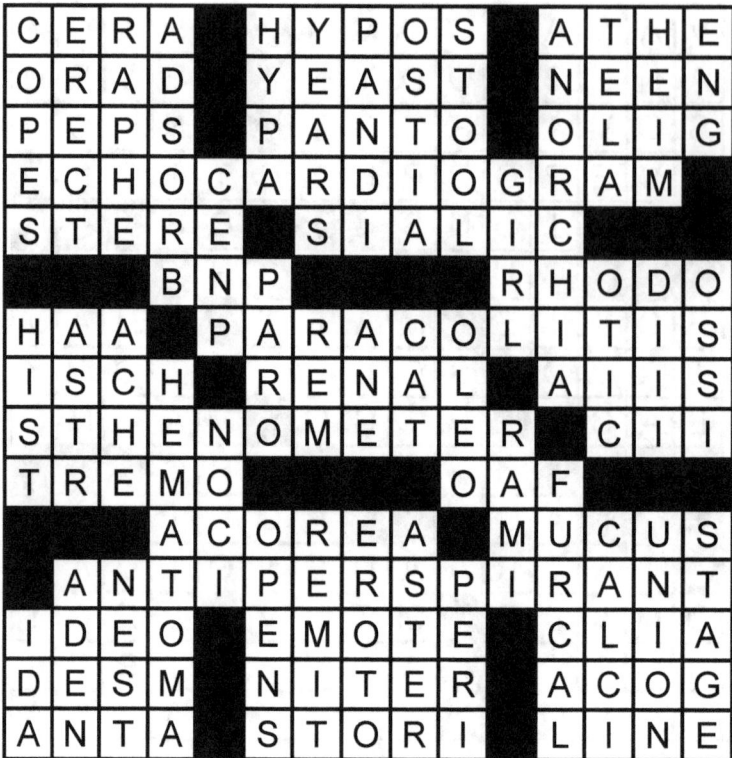

46

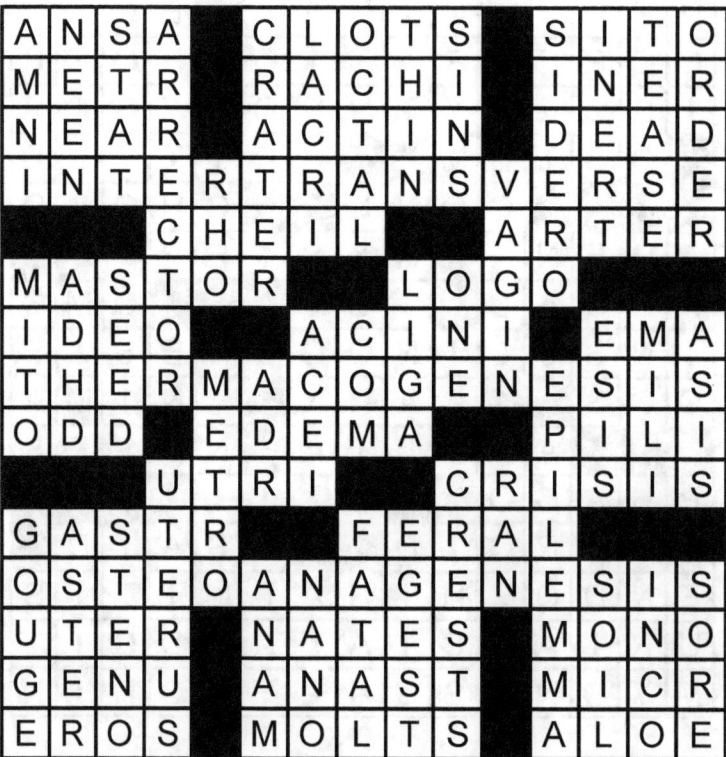

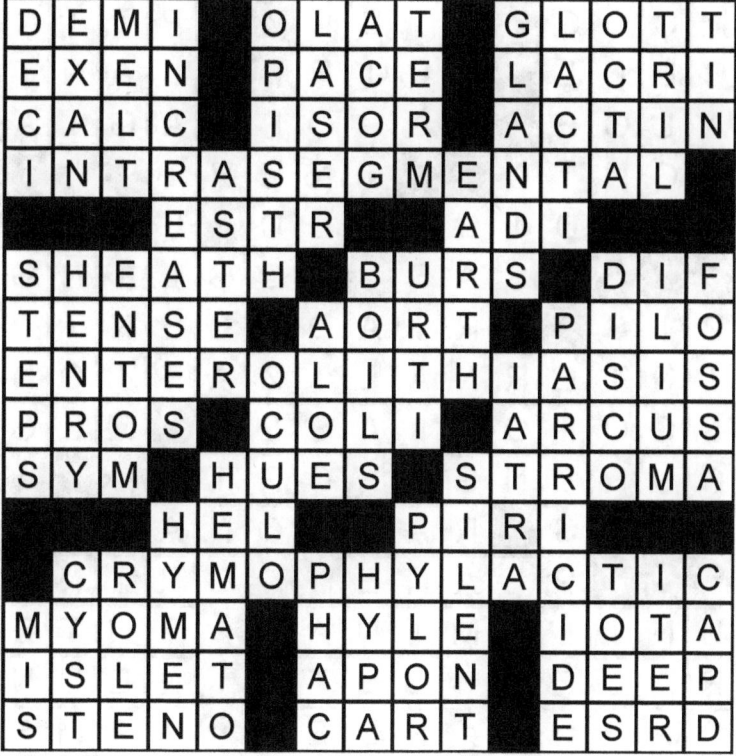

49

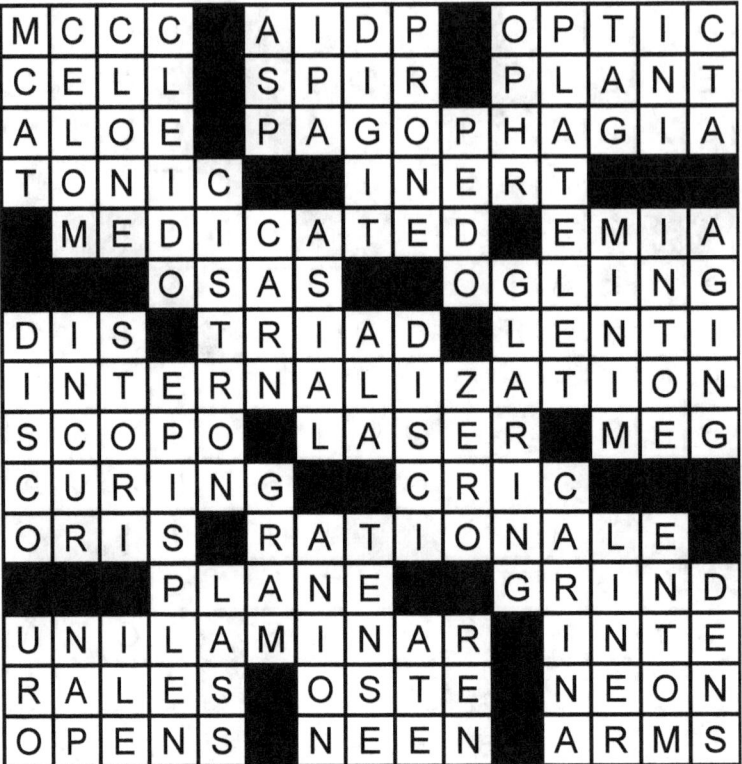

50

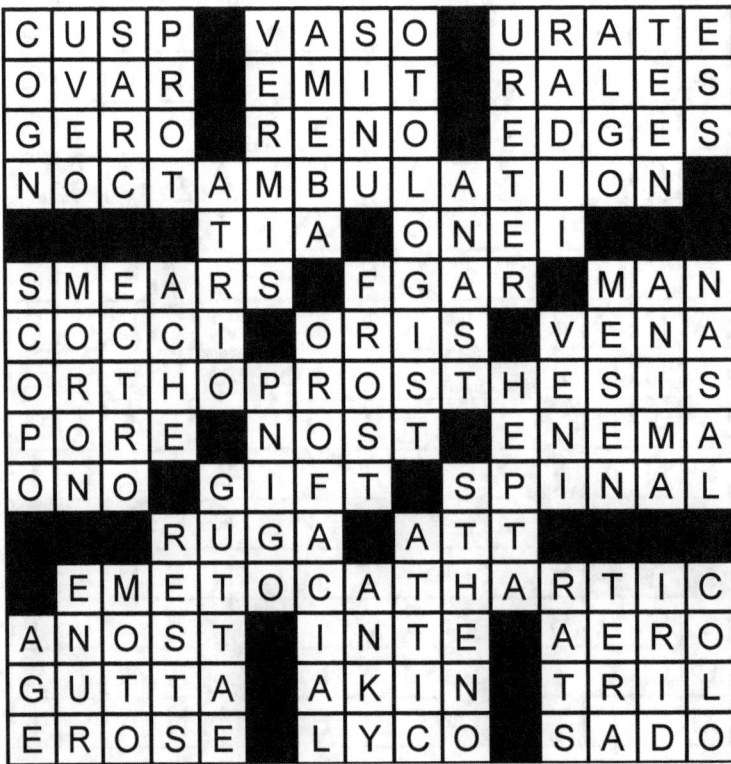

www.ingramcontent.com/pod-product-compliance
Lightning Source LLC
Chambersburg PA
CBHW062227220526
45471CB00009B/3371